Cancer Drugs

DRUGS The Straight Facts

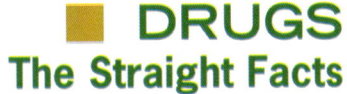

DRUGS
The Straight Facts

Cancer Drugs

Judith Matray-Devoti,
R.Ph., Ph.D

Consulting Editor
David J. Triggle
University Professor
School of Pharmacy and Pharmaceutical Sciences
State University of New York at Buffalo

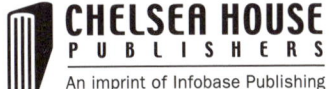

CHELSEA HOUSE
PUBLISHERS
An imprint of Infobase Publishing

Cancer Drugs

Chelsea House
An imprint of Infobase Publishing
132 West 31st Street
New York NY 10001

Library of Congress Cataloging-in-Publication Data

Maltray-Devoti, Judith.
    Cancer drugs / Judith Matray-Devoti.
        p. cm. — (Drugs : the straight facts)
    Includes bibliographical references and index.
    ISBN 0-7910-8554-6 (hardcover)
    1. Cancer—Chemotherapy—Juvenile literature. 2. Antineoplastic
agents—Juvenile literature. I. Title. II. Series.
    RC271. C5M17 2006
    616.99'4061—dc 22   2006020616

Chelsea House books are available at special discounts when purchased in bulk quantities for businesses, associations, institutions, or sales promotions. Please call our Special Sales Department in New York at (212) 967-8800 or (800) 322-8755.

You can find Chelsea House on the World Wide Web at http://www.chelseahouse.com

Text and cover design by Terry Mallon

Printed in the United States of America

Bang EJB 10 9 8 7 6 5 4 3 2 1

This book is printed on acid-free paper.

All links and Web addresses were checked and verified to be correct at the time of publication. Because of the dynamic nature of the Web, some addresses and links may have changed since publication and may no longer be valid.

Table of Contents

Drugs and Their Uses

For many thousands of years, humans have used a variety of agents to cure their ills, promote their well-being, relieve their misery, and control their fertility. Until the beginning of the twentieth century, these agents were all of natural origin, including many of plant origin as well as naturally occurring elements such as arsenic and antimony. The sixteenth century alchemist and physician known as Paracelsus used mercury and arsenic in his treatment of syphilis, worms, and other diseases that were extremely common at that time; his cure rates remain unknown. It is of interest, though, that arsenic trioxide is still used today, albeit in limited fashion, as an anticancer agent, and antimony derivatives are used in the treatment of the tropical disease leishmaniasis.

Our story of modern drug discovery begins with the German physician and scientist Paul Ehrlich. Born in 1854, Ehrlich became interested in the ways in which synthetic dyes, then becoming a major product of the German fine chemical industry, could selectively stain certain tissues and cellular components. He reasoned that such dyes might form the basis for drugs that would selectively interact with diseased cells and organisms. One of Ehrlich's early successes was the arsenical "606"—patented under the name Salvarsan—as a treatment for syphilis. Ehrlich's dream was to create the "magic bullet," a drug that would with absolute specificity target only the diseased cell or the disease-causing organism and not affect healthy tissues and cells. In this he was not successful, but his research did lay the groundwork for the subsequent great discoveries of the twentieth century, including the discovery of the sulfonamide drugs and the antibiotic penicillin. The latter agent saved countless lives during World War II.

From these original advances has come the vast array of drugs that are available to the modern physician. We are increasingly close to Ehrlich's aim of a magic bullet: Drugs can now target very specific molecular defects in a number of cancers, and doctors today have the ability to interrogate the human genome to more effectively match the drug with the patient. In the next one or two decades, it is almost certain that the cost of reading an individual genome will be sufficiently cheap that such "personalized" medicines will become the rule rather than the exception. These drugs do, however, carry very significant costs of both discovery and delivery, thus raising significant social issues of availability and equity of medical treatments.

Despite these current discoveries, it is interesting to note that a very significant fraction of the currently available drugs, notably antibiotics and anticancer agents, are either natural products or are derived from natural products. Such chemicals have been forged in the crucible of evolution and have presumably been derived by nature for very specific biological purposes.

The twenty-first century will continue to produce major advances in medicines and medicine delivery. Nature, however, is also a resilient foe. Diseases and organisms develop resistance to existing drugs so that new molecules must be constantly sought. This is particularly true for anti-infective and anti-cancer agents. Additionally, new and more lethal forms of existing diseases can rapidly develop and with the ease of travel can easily assume pandemic form. Hence the current concerns about avian flu. Also, diseases that have been previously dormant or geographically circumscribed may suddenly break out worldwide. In this way, for instance, an Ebola epidemic would produce many casualties. Finally, there are serious concerns for man-made epidemics through the deliberate spread of existing biological disease agents or through the introduction of a laboratory-manufactured or rejuvenated organism such as smallpox. It is therefore imperative that the search for new medicines continues.

All of us at some point in life will take a medicine, even if it is only aspirin for a headache. For some individuals, drug use will be constant throughout life, as in the current treatment of

AIDS, or will take place only during a certain stage, such as a woman taking hormonal contraceptives during her period of fertility. Quite generally, as we age we will likely be exposed to a variety of medications from childhood vaccines to pain-relieving drugs in a terminal disease. It is not easy to get accurate and understandable knowledge about the drugs that are used to treat diseases. There are, of course, highly specialized volumes and periodicals for the physician and scientist, but these demand a substantial knowledge basis and experience to be fully understood. Advertising on television provides only fleeting information and is usually directed at a single drug; hence the viewer has no means to make a critical or knowledgeable evaluation. The intent of this series of books—*Drugs: The Straight Facts*—is to present to students a readable, intelligent, and accurate description of drugs available for specific diseases, why and how they are used, their limitations, and their side effects. It is our hope that this will provide students with sufficient information to satisfy their immediate needs and give them the background to ask intelligent questions of their health care providers when the need arises.

David J. Triggle, Ph.D.
University Professor
School of Pharmacy and Pharmaceutical Sciences
State University of New York at Buffalo

An in-depth account of drugs and drug discovery can be found in John Mann, *The Elusive Magic Bullet: The Search for the Perfect Drug.* New York: Oxford University Press, 1999.

Introduction

A little over a century ago, oncology—the study of cancer and its treatment—was just getting its start. Some cancers could be treated with surgery, but there were no real drugs for cancer treatment, and a diagnosis of cancer was pretty much a death sentence. Today, oncology is a medical specialty and a detailed education in cancer and its treatments takes years to complete. The diagnosis of cancer has changed from a message of hopelessness to one of increased survival, better quality of life, and, in some cases, even hope for a complete cure.

In the past century, so much has happened to improve cancer therapy that no single book can adequately cover it all. The uses of surgery, radiation, drugs, and other therapies have all made major strides. This book is designed to introduce the reader to some of the drugs that are currently available. Remember that these drugs are only part of the therapies available to any cancer patient, and a course of treatment may include all or some of the other treatment options available. Each type of cancer is best suited to a particular combination of treatments, and each patient's case has its own unique features, requiring a customized approach. Only the basic methods of activity, known risks of use, and unique characteristics of each drug will be described. A doctor should be consulted to put this information into context for any individual patient.

Keep in mind that the information in this book describes the anticancer drugs available in the United States at the time of printing. Some of these drugs may or may not be available in other countries, and some drugs available overseas have not been approved for use in the United States. When they are available overseas, the drugs mentioned in this book may have a different brand name.

1

The Cellular Basis of Cancer

The word *cancer* comes from the Greek word karkinos, for "crab." The physician Hippocrates gave the disease this name around 460 B.C.E. because blood vessels growing through the tumors he observed reminded him of the shape of crab claws. Hippocrates's was not the first written record of the disease. The earliest known description of cancer was found in an ancient Egyptian papyrus written between 3000 and 1500 B.C.E. Clearly, this disease was recognized a long time ago, inspiring many different attempts through the years to explain its cause and to cure it. Early physicians saw that surgery, when possible, often did not stop the return of this devastating disease, so they turned to the natural world for substances to help eliminate cancer regrowth.

As long ago as 300 B.C.E., extracts of ginger root may have been used to treat skin cancers, and the Greek physician Dioscorides (c. 40–90 C.E.) recorded the use of red clover and the autumn crocus, *Colchicum autumnale*, to treat a variety of cancers. These and many other records of attempted therapies eventually led to the development of modern drugs to fight cancer. For example, in 1938, scientists looked further into the ancient Roman use of the autumn crocus and successfully extracted the anticancer drug colchicine.

The search for drugs to treat cancer truly entered the modern era as scientists gained an increased understanding of how cells—especially cancer cells—worked. In this chapter, you will learn about the cell, how cancer cells differ from normal cells, and how cancer drugs take advantage of cellular mechanisms to eliminate cancer cells.

CELL STRUCTURES AND THEIR FUNCTIONS

Although some groups of cells in the body have specialized characteristics, all cells share basic structures that are necessary for performing the same basic functions. Cancer cells share these structures, too, but the way they control their functions and respond to environmental changes differs from the methods that normal cells use. Cancer cells will be discussed later; normal cell properties are described here first.

The cell is surrounded by a flexible, permeable membrane that organizes the cell's structure and controls its interaction with its environment. The membrane is a fluid environment with specialized proteins suspended in it. These proteins respond to chemical signals from both inside and outside the cell. Inside the cell, the **cytoplasm** (a watery fluid) surrounds a number of important structures, or **organelles** (Figure 1.1):

- **nucleus**—where the cell's genetic material is stored in the form of a molecule called **DNA** (deoxyribonucleic acid). DNA defines how a cell functions during its lifespan, how and when it will divide, and how long the cell will live.

- **mitochondria**—these organelles convert nutrients into usable energy.

- **lysosomes**—cellular digestive enzymes are found in these membrane sacs in the cytoplasm. They are used to process materials for elimination from the cells, and even clean up the remains of the cell itself when it dies.

- **endoplasmic reticulum**—this structure is important to protein and DNA synthesis (production). Cells manufacture proteins to control almost all their functions and to affect the function of other cells in their environment. **Ribosomes** are small structures often found on the endoplasmic reticulum. They translate information from the nucleus that is necessary for manufacturing proteins or DNA.

- **microtubules**—these are hollow, tubular filaments made of a protein called **tubulin**. They create some of the structural elements of the cell. They play an important role in separating the two cells formed during cell division. **Centrioles** are specialized microtubules that organize the division of cells.

THE CELL CYCLE AND ITS PHASES

Cancer is generally defined as a growth or tumor that results from abnormal and uncontrolled cell division. Normal cells of the body, with a few exceptions, constantly undergo cell division as old and injured cells die off and are replaced. The process of controlled growth and death of normal cells is referred to as **homeostasis**, and its goal is to maintain a healthy balance in the life processes of the cells, tissues, and organs of the body.

To achieve this goal, cell growth and division occurs in a process called the cell cycle, and its steps are carefully controlled by a variety of genetic and molecular feedback mechanisms. In cancer cells, any one or several of these mechanisms malfunction, allowing the cells' growth to proceed unchecked.

The cell cycle is an orderly, four-stage process. The cell starts the cycle when it is engaged in its normal functions. It eventually prepares to make a copy of itself by entering a phase in which the the cell's DNA—its genetic material—replicates, resulting in duplicate genetic material. The cell returns to its normal functions for a while before entering the final phase, when the cytoplasm and duplicate genetic material separates producing two identical cells.

Normal cells follow the steps of the cell cycle in an orderly fashion. Cancer cells also follow these steps, but they bypass the

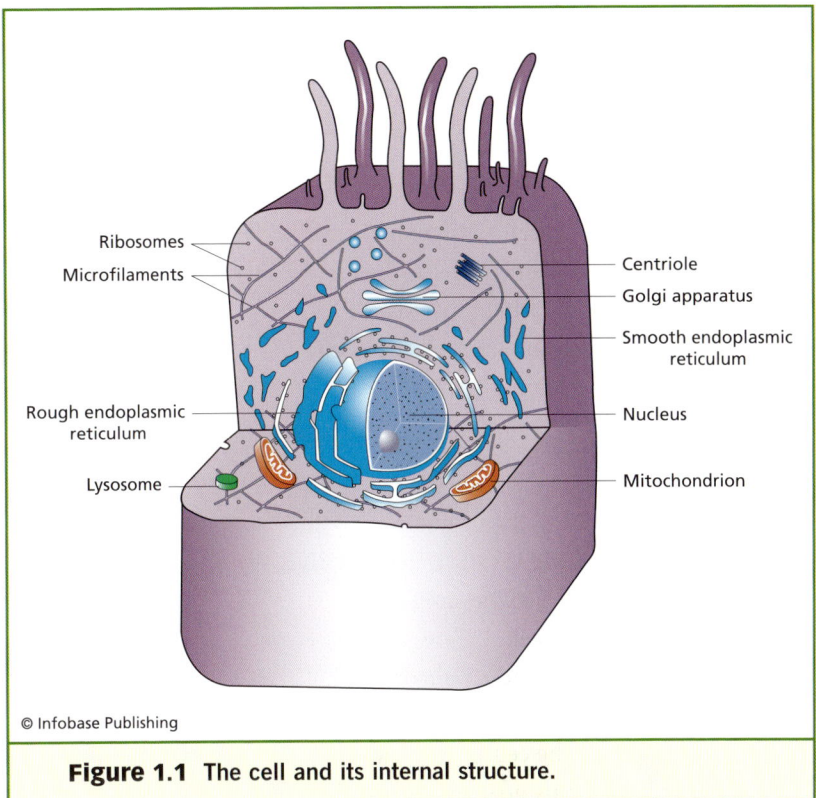

© Infobase Publishing

Figure 1.1 The cell and its internal structure.

controls that keep too many of them from entering the cycle at once and that make them die off when they should.

IMPORTANT FEATURES OF TUMOR GROWTH: CELL DIVISION

Cancer cells do not stop dividing the way normal cells do. There are four ways that cancer cells differ from normal cells that cause them to grow uncontrollably:

1. Normal cells require external growth factors to enter the cell cycle. External growth factors are substances from the surrounding environment that trigger division. Cancer

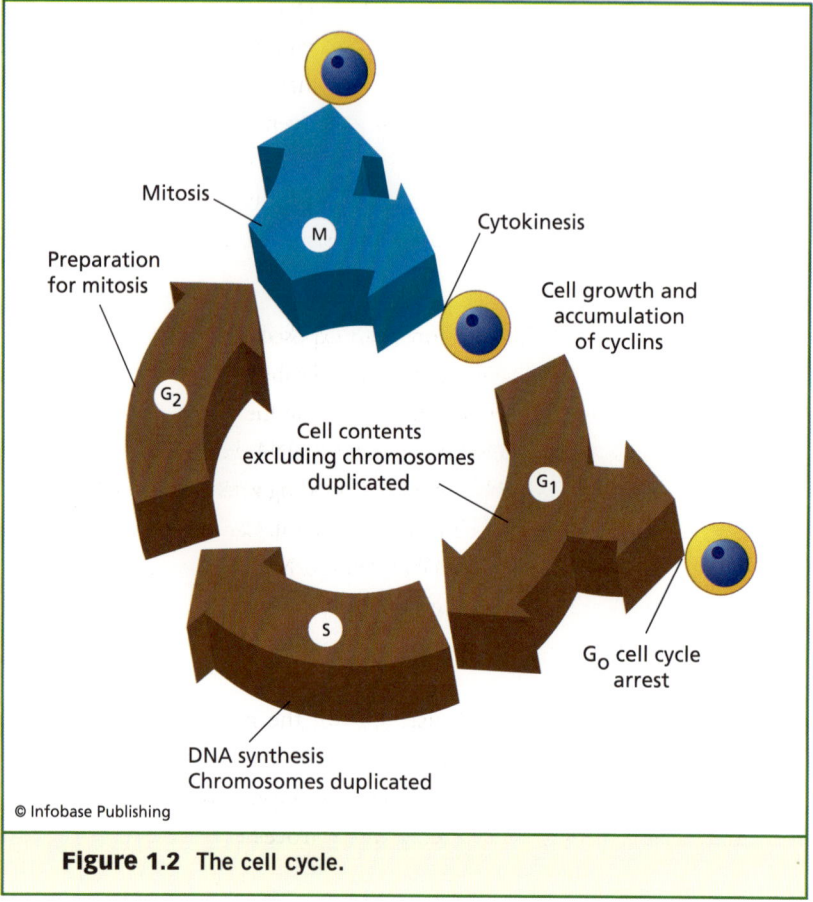

Mitosis

Cytokinesis

Preparation
for mitosis

Cell growth and
accumulation
of cyclins

M

G_2

Cell contents
excluding chromosomes
duplicated

G_1

S

G_0 cell cycle
arrest

DNA synthesis
Chromosomes duplicated

© Infobase Publishing

Figure 1.2 The cell cycle.

cells live independently of these growth factors, so they
continually divide.

2. Normal cells limit their division when they come into
   contact with other cells. Cancer cells continue to grow
   even after touching other cells, resulting in an accumulat-
   ing mass of cells.

3. Normal cells eventually die, to be replaced by new ones.
   Each time a mature cell divides, a structure called a
   telomere at the end of the DNA shortens. When the

telomere is gone, the cell can no longer divide. Young, immature cells have an enzyme called **telomerase** that replaces the telomere until the cell matures. Mature cells stop producing telomerase, so they eventually die off in a process of programmed cell death called **apoptosis**. Cancer cells, on the other hand, constantly produce telomerase. This allows them to avoid apoptosis and keep dividing endlessly.

4. The DNA of all cells is constantly exposed to destructive energies, like radiation from the sun, and substances, like waste materials from the surrounding cells, in the course of a cell's life, but normal cells can repair most DNA damage. Normal cells become unable to continue dividing when their DNA is damaged beyond their ability to repair it. Cancer cells, however, are not limited by DNA damage. Not only do they continue to divide when their DNA is damaged, but they pass on this genetic damage to future generations of cancer cells.

Each of these characteristics, from the many genetic and molecular controls of the cell cycle to the growth mechanisms that go wrong in cancer cells provide an opportunity for a drug to interfere with the damaged growth processes of cancer.

HOW CANCER DRUGS WORK

All cancer drugs ultimately have the same action: They interfere with or stop the growth of living cells. How they achieve this goal differs by the cellular functions on which each drug acts. The same characteristics that contribute to cell growth can be used against the cell, and chemotherapy takes advantage of these opportunities. The actions of cancer drugs fall into several broad categories.

Targeting cell function and molecular synthesis

Cells are continually processing nutrients and synthesizing new molecules from the products of nutrient **metabolism**. Some

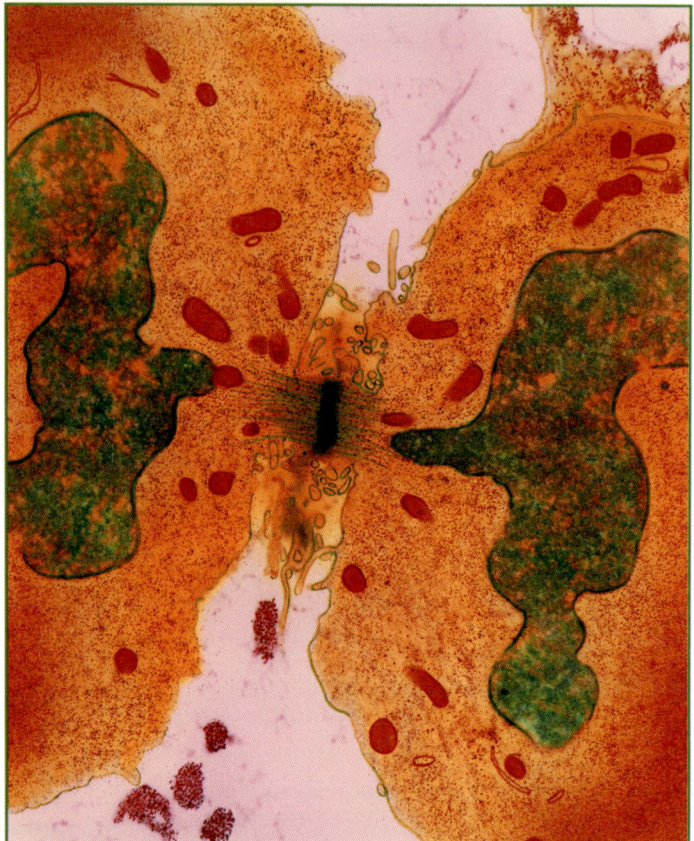

Figure 1.3   Dividing cancer cell. Colored transmission electron (TEM) of a section through a cancer cell undergoing mitotic cell division. The cell is in telophase, the last stage of mitosis. Nuclear envelopes have formed around the duplicate chromosome sets creating two nuclei (green). The cytoplasm (orange) contains mitochondria (red). The two daughter cells are connected by a narrow cytoplasmic bridge (at center). © Quest/Photo Researchers, Inc.

classes of cancer drugs work because their chemical structure mimics some nutrient or essential molecule so closely that the cell incorporates the drug into its processes. Like a wrench thrown into the gears of a machine, a drug that imperfectly matches the molecule that the cell needs interferes with its functions, and eventually causes cell death.

Altering cell signaling and organization

Normal cells send many chemical signals to structures within the cell and to other cells in the body to start and stop the processes that sustain life. The cell cycle, for instance, depends on the coordinated delivery and receipt of numerous signals. Another example involves the body's immune system. Normally, the body's immune defenses detect cells that are foreign to the body, such as bacteria, or finds badly damaged cells, and send signals to immune cells to remove the foreign invader or the injured cell that cannot start apoptosis. Cancer cells often do not trigger an appropriate immune response, so some drugs have been developed to trick the immune system into taking action against cancerous cells.

Affecting cell surface receptors

Specialized proteins embedded in the cell membrane, called **receptors**, continually latch on to specific chemicals in the environment. Receptors change some cellular functions when they bind to passing chemical signals. For example, some chemicals stimulate the cell to grow, others can make the cell speed up its functions, and other chemicals can signal the cell that it is time to die. Some cancers continue their growth because they become very sensitive to growth signals, or because they become insensitive to the signals that normally stop cell growth. Certain cancer drugs can block growth signals from attaching to cell receptors, cutting the cell off from its growth triggers.

Changing the cancer cell environment

In another strategy related to cell signaling, some cancer drugs act to change the production or availability of specific molecules in the body so that cancer cell receptors do not receive certain chemical signals. For instance, some cancers rely on the presence of normal body hormones to continue growing and dividing. Blocking the body's production of these hormones stops the cancer from growing.

THE BEST WAY TO ADMINISTER A CANCER DRUG

Ideally, drugs that are given to eliminate cancer cells would only come into contact with cancer cells, to protect normal cells from damage. In practice, this is rarely possible. While research continues to look for ways to selectively deliver drugs

HOW DO CANCER DRUGS KNOW TO ATTACK ONLY CANCER CELLS?

One problem with cancer drugs is that they do not know to attack only cancer cells. A drug in the body circulates and contacts most body tissues and cells. The reason that chemotherapy does not kill all the normal cells is mostly because of two useful cell characteristics:

1. Normal cells have repair mechanisms that can help them recover from damage.

2. Cancer cells generally cannot repair themselves effectively.

Even though they can repair themselves, some normal cells die from exposure to cancer drugs, or cannot function well even after repair. Normal cells that divide often are most at risk. These would include the cells that line the stomach and intestines, hair follicle cells, and bone marrow cells. This accounts for many of the bad side effects (adverse effects) of cancer drugs, including nausea, vomiting, hair loss, and other problems. Modern therapy with cancer drugs is usually given with treatments to prevent or manage many of these adverse effects.

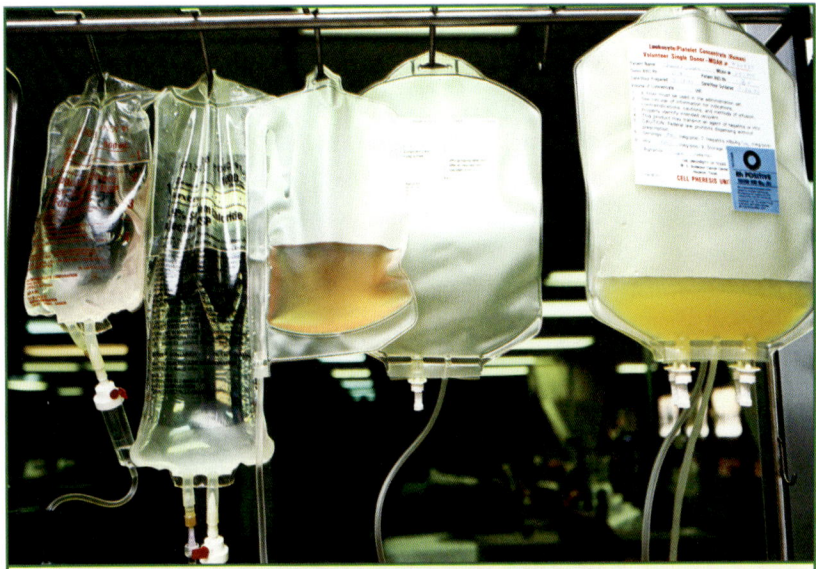

Figure 1.4 Chemicals for cancer treatment. © Bernard Annebicque/CORBIS SYGMA

to their intended targets, most cancer drugs today are circulated throughout the body. Like many other drugs, cancer drugs may be given orally (by mouth) as capsules or tablets. Once in the digestive system, they are absorbed and eventually travel throughout the body in the bloodstream. Most chemotherapy, however, is given by **intravenous** (in a vein) injection, sending the drug directly into the bloodstream. When this is done by slowly dripping a drug solution into a vein, it is called **intravenous infusion**.

Since there are few options for changing the way cancer drugs are introduced to the body, other methods have been created to improve the drugs' impact on cancer cells. Most cancer drugs are dosed in **regimens**, or patterns of administration, that are timed both to affect cancer cells in the vulnerable phases of their growth cycle and to allow the noncancerous cells of the body to recover. Regimens are also devised to

SARCOMA, LEUKEMIA, MYELOMA, CARCINOMA—WHY ALL THE DIFFERENT WORDS FOR CANCER?

Cancers can be classified in two ways: by the type of tissue from which they arise or by the location in the body from which they start to grow. The first way is known as classification by histology and is defined internationally. The second method of classification is not very useful to doctors, but the general public may find it easier to talk about cancers as being in the breast, or lung.

There are five major histological classifications:

Carcinoma—These cancers grow from epithelial tissue, which is tissue that makes up the outer and inner lining of the body. Carcinomas account for as much as 90 percent of all cancers.

Sarcoma—These cancers develop in supportive and structural body tissues, like bones, muscles, tendons, cartilage, and fat.

Myeloma—These cancers develop in the plasma cells of the bone marrow. These are cells that produce some of the proteins that circulate in the bloodstream.

Leukemia—These cancers are also called liquid cancers or blood cancers. They start in the bone marrow. They cause an overproduction of white blood cells that do not reach their mature form, but they can also cause cancerous growth of red blood cells.

Lymphoma—These cancers originate in the organs and tissues of the lymphatic system, including lymph nodes, spleen, or tonsils. Since lymph vessels circulate all through the body, a lymphoma may develop in the lymph system of any organ, such as the stomach, breast, or brain.

Table 1.1 Cancer Drug Classes and their Characteristics

Class	Characteristic
Alkylating agents	Share a similar chemical structure
Antimetabolites	Target cell metabolism
Natural products	Derived from plant source
Hormones and hormone antagonists	Mimic the body's hormones or block them
Molecularly targeted agents	Target particular cellular chemicals
Biological response modifiers	Affect the body's immune system response
Miscellaneous agents	Variety of mechanisms, structures, and sources

combine several cancer drugs. Combination therapy tries to use drugs that each affects a different cell function to weaken cancer cells as much as possible. In a variation of combination therapy, called adjunct therapy, the combination regimen is administered before or after surgery or **radiation therapy**. The regimen is timed to produce the greatest therapeutic benefit with the least damage to the patient.

Classes of Cancer Drugs

There are many logical ways to group cancer drugs to make them easier to understand. Some of these categories group chemically similar drugs together, some group the drugs based on the cell functions they target, and other categories group the drugs by origin.

2

Alkylating Agents

The first modern cancer chemotherapy agents were discovered as a result of the development of chemical warfare agents during World War I (1914–1918). On December 2, 1943, during World War II, German bombers attacked American tankers and munitions ships in Bari Harbor off the southeastern coast of Italy. Sixteen ships sank and four more were damaged, setting off at least two major explosions. Hundreds of men were pulled out of the oily, burning waters.

The oil-covered survivors appeared fine at first, but soon began to complain of internal problems, stinging eyes, and skin lesions. Four died that day, nine the next day, and by the end of the month, 83 of the 617 survivors were dead.

One of the ships had been secretly carrying 100 tons of mustard gas. This chemical was used during World War I as a weapon to cause severe blistering of the skin, eyes, and lungs of soldiers exposed to it. It gets its name from the mustard-like smell of the impure chemical; once purified, it is odorless and colorless. Although most of the mustard gas in the Bari Harbor incident burned off in the fires following the explosions, some of it dissolved in the floating oil, causing the only American mustard gas casualties of World War II.

Autopsies showed that the bone marrow and **lymphatic** tissues of these men were damaged by the gas. As a result, they produced fewer red blood cells (**erythrocytes**), white blood cells (**leukocytes**), and immune system cells (**lymphocytes**) than normal. This observation led researchers in 1943 to use **nitrogen mustards** to treat Hodgkin's disease and lymphocytic **lymphoma**, cancers related to the overproduction of cells from the bone marrow and lymphatic tissues.

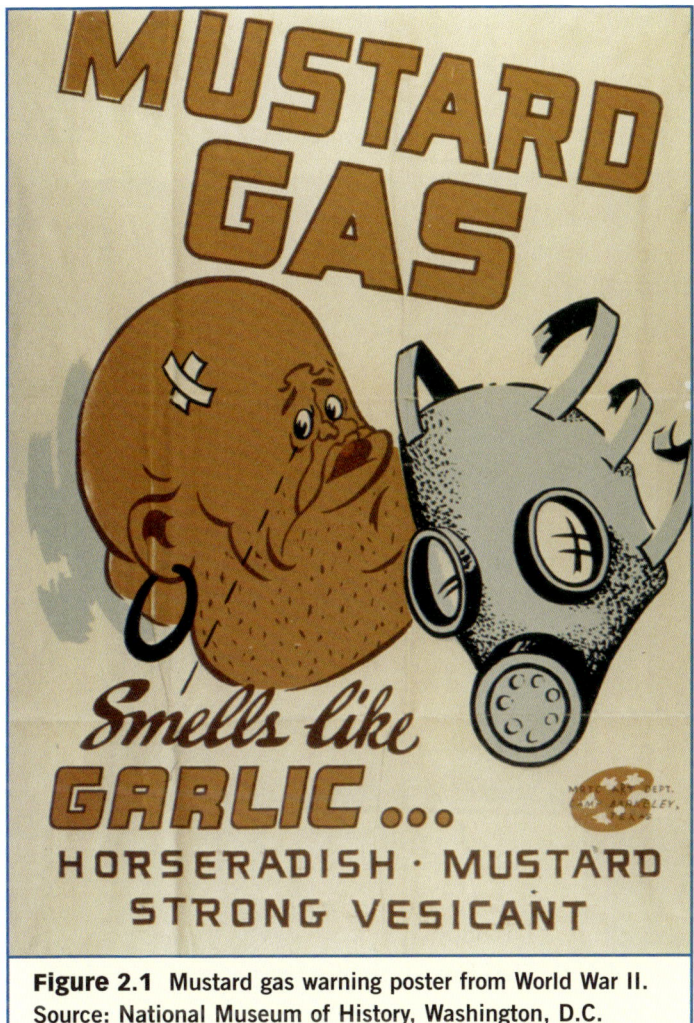

Figure 2.1 Mustard gas warning poster from World War II.
Source: National Museum of History, Washington, D.C.

Because of the secret nature of the wartime weapons program, the results of this medical research were not published until 1946.

Initial results were very exciting, because the drug caused a dramatic regression of advanced lymphomas, but unfortunately, the tumors always returned. Despite the disappointing lack of a cure, research with chemicals related to mustard gas, continued, eventually leading to successful advances with combined cancer therapies in the 1960s. Research into the nitrogen mustards gave rise to a whole family of chemically related compounds used to treat a variety of cancers. Today, these **alkylating agents** continue to be the most widely used anticancer drugs.

DRUGS IN THE CATEGORY OF ALKYLATING AGENTS

The earliest members of this class were called nitrogen mustards, since they all shared part of the chemical structure of the original chemical warfare agent known as mustard gas. The following Figure 2.2 demonstrates this structure and the similarities between the first alkylating agents.

Later alkylating agents departed more and more from these early chemical structures, but they successfully acted on cancer through similar mechanisms. Table 2.1 summarizes these agents.

HOW DO ALKYLATING AGENTS WORK?

DNA is like a paired string of pearls, and each pearl is a molecule called a **base**. The string is built from a sugar called "deoxyribose" and from phosphorous and oxygen groups called "phosphates." Attached to the deoxyribose molecules in the "string" are four kinds of nitrogen-containing bases or "pearls": adenine (A), guanine (G), cytosine (C), and thymine (T). These bases can be sorted into two groups: purines and pyrimidines. Adenine and guanine are purines, which are larger than the pyrimidines cytosine and thymine. There are other purines and pyrimidines that are used as building blocks for other molecules in a cell, but these are the only ones that are used to create DNA strands.

The two strands of DNA are joined by bonds between the complementary bases of purines and pyrimidines. The purine adenine (A) always bonds to the pyrimidine thymine (T) on the opposite strand. Guanine (G) always bonds to cytosine

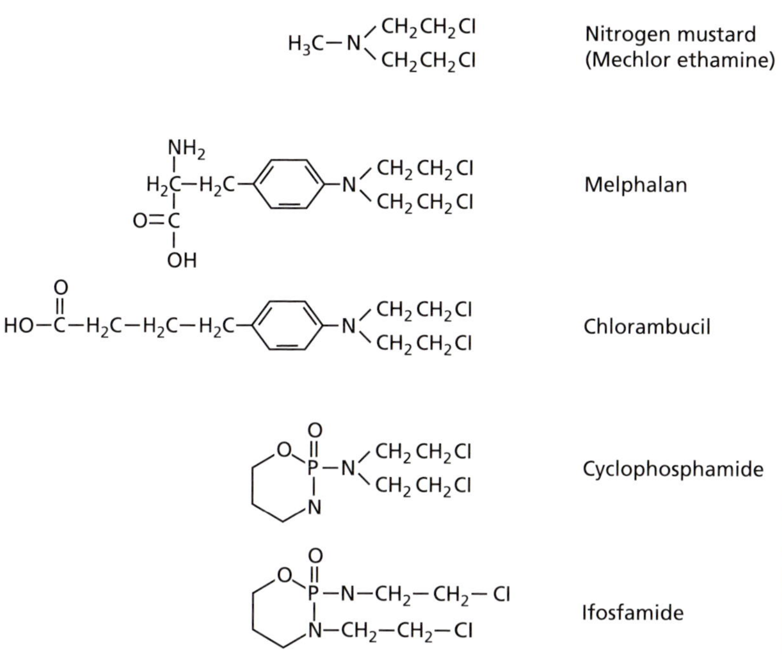

Figure 2.2 Chemical structures of some early alkylating agents. Note their similarity to the first agent in the class, nitrogen mustard (mechlorethamine).

(C). This specific bonding, or pairing, is critical for the formation of stable DNA molecules that control the life processes of cells.

Groups of paired bases form genes. The genes act like codes that tell the cell how to function.

Alkylating agents work directly on DNA to prevent cancer cells from reproducing. These agents are active in all phases of the cell cycle. There are three ways that alkylating agents interfere with the function of DNA:

1. In the first mechanism, the alkylating agent attaches short organic molecules called alkyl groups to DNA bases. This

Table 2.1 The Alkylating Agents

Category	Generic name (alternative name)	Trademark name (manufacturer or distributor)
Nitrogen mustards	Mechlorethamine	Mustargen® (Merck)
	Melphalan (L-PAM, phenylalanine mustard)	Alkeran® (GlaxoSmithKline)
	Chlorambucil	Leukeran® (GlaxoSmithKline)
	Cyclophosphamide	Cytoxan® (Bristol-Myers Squibb)
		Neosar® (Sicor Labs)
	Ifosfamide	Ifex® (Bristol-Myers Squibb)
Ethyleneimines and methylenimines	Hexamethylmelamine (altretamine)	Hexalen® (MGI Pharma)
	Thiotepa	(generic; produced by various manufacturers)
Alkyl sulfonates	Busulfan	Myleran® (GlaxoSmithKline)
		Busulfex® (ESP Pharma)
Nitrosoureas	Carmustine (BCNU)	BiCNU® (Bristol-Myers Squibb)
	Lomustine (CCNU)	Gliadel® (Guilford Pharmaceuticals)
		CEENU® (Bristol-Myers Squibb)
	Streptozocin	Zanosar® (Sicor Pharmaceuticals)
Tetrazines	Dacarbazine (DTIC)	DTIC-DOME® (Bayer Pharmaceuticals)
	Temozolomide	Temodar® (Schering-Plough)
Metal salts	Cisplatin	Platinol®, Platinol-AQ® (Bristol-Myers Squibb)
	Carboplatin	Paraplatin® (Bristol-Myers Squibb)
	Oxaliplatin	Eloxatin® (Sanofi Aventis)

Many of these agents are also available in generic form through various manufacturers.

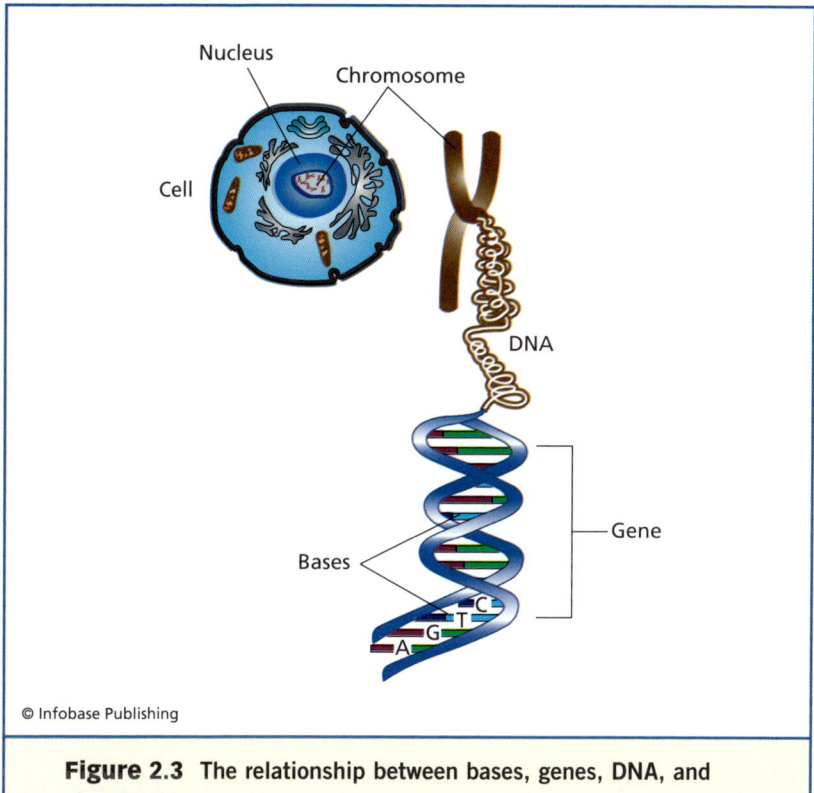

Figure 2.3 The relationship between bases, genes, DNA, and chromosomes.

results in the DNA being broken apart by the cell's own repair enzymes when they try to replace the damaged bases (see Figure 2.4).

2. Alkylating agents cause atoms in the DNA molecule to bond differently from the way they normally do. This prevents the two strands of DNA from temporarily separating the way they should when the process of cellular reproduction begins (see Figure 2.5).

3. Alkylating agents cause the bases in the DNA molecule to pair up incorrectly. This leads to mutations that impair or destroy the cell's function (see Figure 2.6).

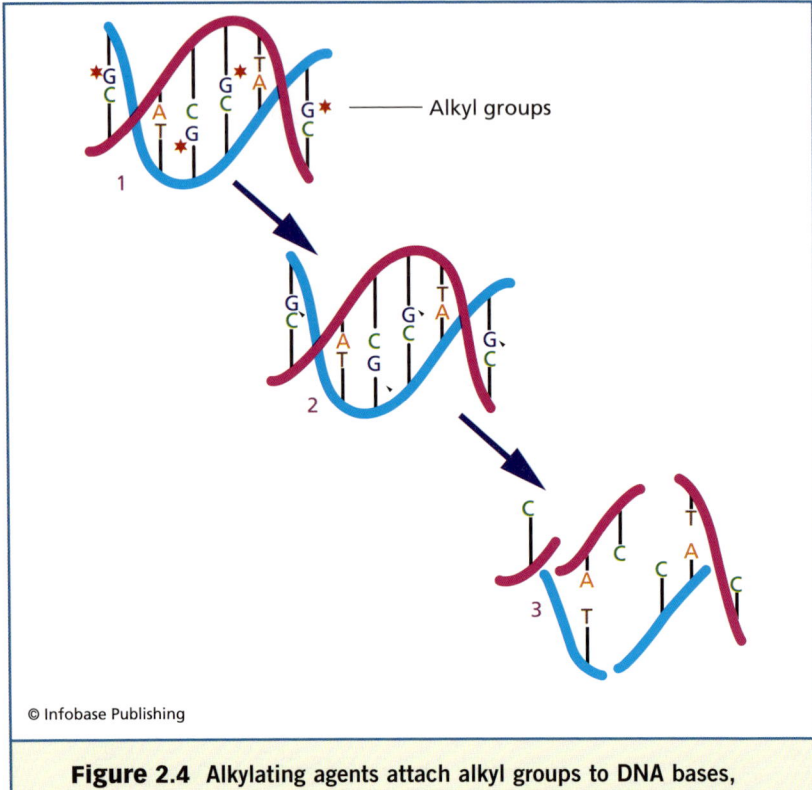

Alkyl groups

Figure 2.4 Alkylating agents attach alkyl groups to DNA bases, causing them to break apart.

Alkylating agents are approved to treat **leukemias** that are **chronic**; non-Hodgkin's lymphoma; Hodgkin's disease; multiple **myeloma**; and lung, breast, ovarian, brain, and other cancers.

NITROGEN MUSTARDS

There are several nitrogen mustards in use as cancer treatments, including mechlorethamine, melphalan, chlorambucil, cyclophosphamide, and ifosfamide. Mechlorethamine was the prototype for the alkylating agents. It is not often used today except in combination regimens for the treatment of Hodgkin's disease. It is sometimes used **topically** (on the skin)

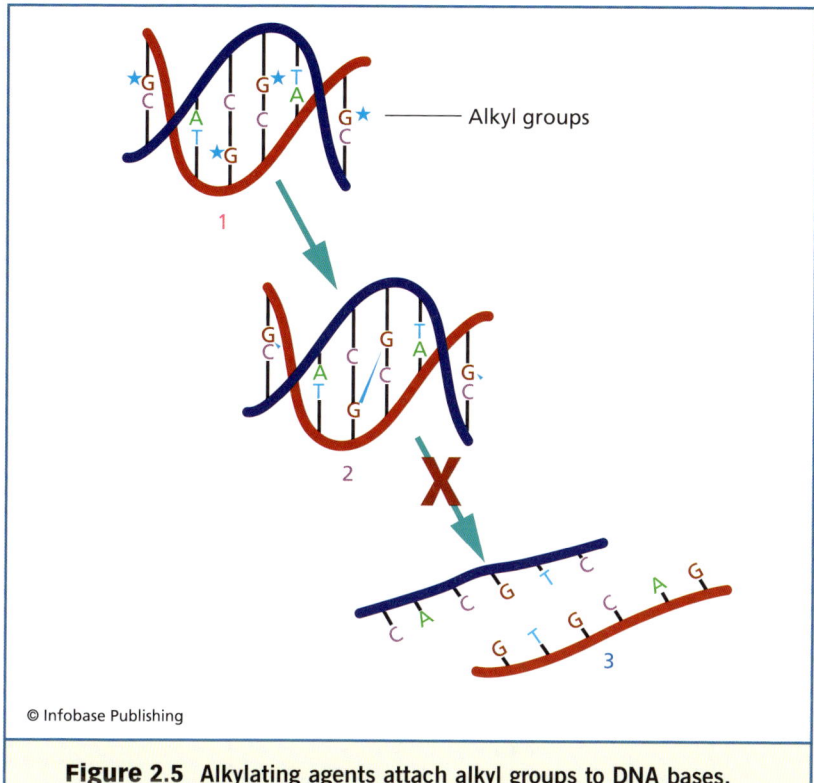

Alkyl groups

Figure 2.5 Alkylating agents attach alkyl groups to DNA bases, causing them to bond differently.

to treat mycosis fungoides, a slowly progressing lymphoma that causes red patches on the skin that eventually develop into tumors. The most important adverse effect of mechlorethamine is **myelosuppression** (suppression of the bone marrow's production of many types of blood cells). It can also cause blood clots and injury to the vein at the time of injection.

Melphalan and chlorambucil were created in the hope of synthesizing drugs that would act more specifically on tumor cells, sparing normal cells. Although that goal was not entirely realized, both of these drugs are often used in the treatment of several cancers. Melphalan is used to treat multiple myeloma and ovarian cancer—either as a single agent or in combination

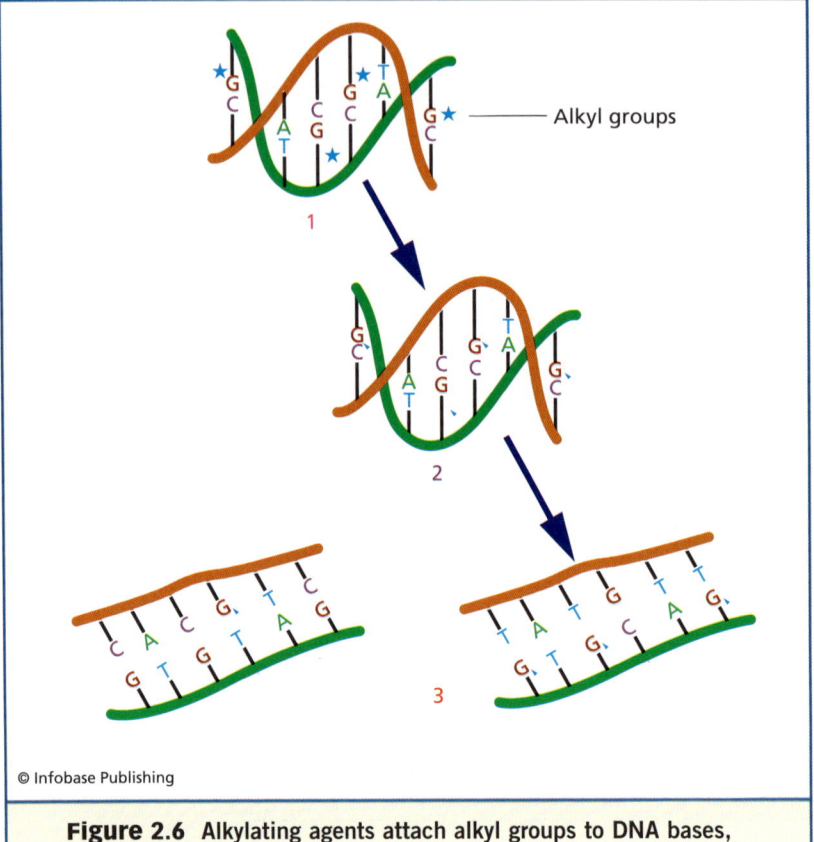

Alkyl groups

Figure 2.6 Alkylating agents attach alkyl groups to DNA bases, causing them to mispair.

with other cancer drugs. Chlorambucil is used to treat chronic lymphocytic leukemia, and **malignant** lymphomas. Like mechlorethamine, melphalan and chlorambucil cause myelo-suppression as their most common adverse effect.

Cyclophosphamide is the most widely used alkylating agent and may actually be the most widely used cancer drug. It was the first cancer agent developed to be administered as a **prodrug**: a drug that required the body's metabolism to change the drug to its active form. It quickly demonstrated that it worked against a variety of cancers, and the diseases for which

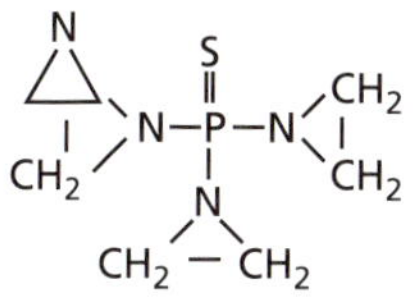

© Infobase Publishing

Figure 2.7 Ethyleneimine (thiotepa) and methyleneimine (altreatamine) are both chemically similar to alkylating agents.

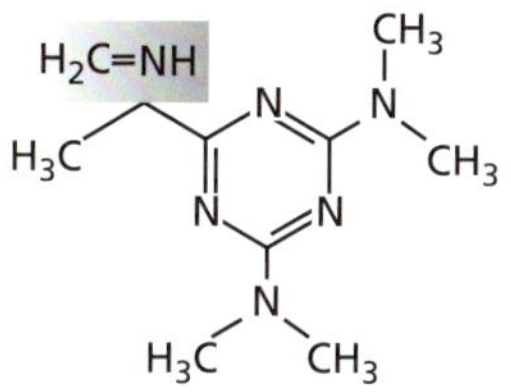

it is currently approved include malignant lymphomas, multiple myeloma, leukemias, advanced mycosis fungoides, neuroblastoma, adenocarcinoma of the ovary, retinoblastoma, and breast **carcinoma**. Myelosuppression and alopecia are important adverse effects of this drug, which can also cause damage to the heart muscle when used in high doses.

Ifosfamide, like cyclophosphamide, is a prodrug that works against a variety of cancers. It is approved for use in the treatment of germ cell testicular cancer and bone and soft tissue **sarcomas**. This drug is excreted from the body in the urine, and can cause hemorrhagic cystitis, a condition in which the lining of the bladder becomes inflamed and bleeds. To prevent this, a drug called mesna is given prior to or along with the ifosfamide dose.

ETHYLENEIMINES AND METHYLENEIMINES

The ethyleneimines and methyleneimines, which include thiotepa and altretamine, incorporate a simple, nitrogen-based

WHAT IS AN APPROVED USE?

In 1906, the U.S. government passed the Food and Drug Act, which prohibited interstate commerce in misbranded foods and drugs. This happened at a time when sanitary inspections of meatpacking plants were poor in quality, if they were done at all, and when government oversight of drug production was nonexistent. The act was meant to improve these conditions, but unfortunately it did not define the necessary guidelines for oversight, nor did it empower any government body to take legal action. In 1937, the maker of Elixir Sulfanilamide substituted diethylene glycol—antifreeze—for a safer solvent and killed 107 patients, most of them children. Partly in response to this tragedy, the government passed the Food, Drug, and Cosmetic Act of 1938. This act allowed the Food and Drug Administration (FDA) to take action against companies that could not prove the safety of the drugs they sold. Over the years, the FDA's role in the regulation of drugs sold in the United States has expanded. Drugs are not only tested for safety, but companies also have to prove that a drug is effective before they can sell the product.

Although a drug manufacturer can only advertise the use of a drug for its approved indication (FDA-approved use), a doctor is free to use his or her professional experience and judgment in the use of any approved drug. This means that a doctor may prescribe a drug for a disease that it is not approved for, or at a dose different from the approved one. This is a common practice and a necessary one. No company is capable of testing a cancer drug for use with every possible cancer. Doctors who are familiar with the way these drugs work and who understand the nature of the cancer they are treating can determine which drugs will be effective against the disease. They share this information with other doctors, even publishing their observations so that patients can benefit from the best possible treatments.

molecule into their overall chemical structure, while remaining similar to the rest of the alkylating agents. Thiotepa is similar to mechlorethamine, but does not irritate the tissues it contacts. It is approved for use in the treatment of specific cancers of the breast, ovary, and bladder. It has been effective in the treatment of some lymphomas, but newer treatments are preferred over thiotepa.

Although altretamine is chemically similar to the other alkylating agents, its specific mechanism of action is not well understood. It shares the typical adverse effects of this class of drugs, including myelosuppression. In addition, it often causes sensory **neuropathy** (degeneration of the nerves that sense touch, temperature, or pain) in the hands and feet. Taking vitamin B_6 (pyridoxine) can help avoid the nerve damage, but may reduce the drug's effectiveness against cancer.

ALKYL SULFONATE

The alkyl sulfonates differ in chemical structure from the rest of the alkylating agents by including a group of atoms that contain sulfur and oxygen. Busulfan is currently the only alkyl sulfonate used as a cancer treatment.

Busulfan was manufactured in an attempt to create an alkylating agent that would be less toxic than mechlorethamine. It has a limited range of activity against cancer, and is indicated only for the **palliative** (easing symptoms without curing) treatment of chronic myelogenous leukemia. Unfortunately, myelosuppression is its most common adverse event, and it can occasionally cause a fatal liver disorder.

NITROSOUREAS

Nitrosoureas include carmustine (BCNU), lomustine (CCNU), and streptozocin. They have a chemical structure derived from the nitrogen mustards.

Carmustine is used to treat multiple myeloma and certain lymphomas when given by injection. A special form of

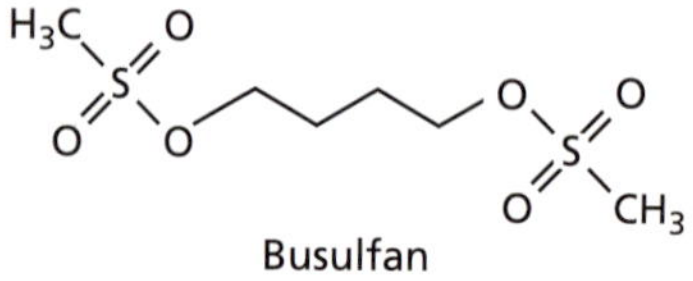

Busulfan

© Infobase Publishing

Figure 2.8 Busulfan contains a chain of carbon atoms connected to the oxygen-sulfur group.

carmustine is used to treat brain tumors. A thin wafer of a polymer material is saturated with carmustine and the wafer is implanted directly into the brain near the tumor. The drug slowly seeps out of the wafer and is absorbed by the tumor cells. In its injectable form, carmustine often causes delayed myelosuppression that may be prolonged. At high doses, it commonly causes serious **toxicity** (a poisonous effect) that affects the lungs, brain, or liver. These adverse effects are avoided by using the wafers instead of the injectable form.

Lomustine is used to treat lung and kidney cancers, certain lymphomas, and brain tumors. Like carmustine, it commonly causes delayed and prolonged myelosuppression.

Streptozocin is approved to treat a type of cancer of the pancreas. It sometimes causes serious **renal** (referring to the kidneys) toxicity, along with the usual effects of the nitrogen mustards.

TETRAZINES

The tetrazines, which include dacarbazine (DTIC) and temozolomide, were synthesized in the laboratory from the structure of the nitrogen mustards. Like the nitrogen mustards, they are effective alkylating agents.

Dacarbazine is one of the few cancer drugs that work against the skin cancer melanoma. In addition to myelosuppression, it can cause a liver toxicity that is sometimes slow to develop and may be fatal.

Temozolomide is available in capsule form to treat brain tumors. Myelosuppression, nausea, and vomiting are common side effects in patients who take this drug.

METAL SALTS

The metal salts include cisplatin, carboplatin, and oxaliplatin. Although these drugs are alkylating agents, they do not share a chemical structure with the nitrogen mustards. Instead, they get their ability to interfere with the structure of DNA from the existence of an atom of platinum in their molecule. The platinum is highly reactive and readily forms bonds with parts of the DNA molecule. Remember that like other cancer drugs, these alkylating agents will affect all cells in the body.

Cisplatin was the first of the platinum compounds found to be active against cancer. This drug may be best known as being part of the treatment regimen for Lance Armstrong, the champion bicycle rider who not only won the grueling Tour de France seven times, but also won his fight against testicular cancer. It is approved for use in advanced testicular, ovarian,

SIDE EFFECT OR ADVERSE EFFECT?

Strictly speaking, a side effect is any unwanted effect of a drug, whether it is harmful or not. An adverse effect is not only unwanted, but harmful. When the U.S. Food and Drug Administration (FDA) evaluates a drug for efficacy and safety, it weighs the good and the bad before approving or rejecting the drug. Although all the adverse effects listed for some of these drugs may be frightening, the drugs' benefits outweigh the bad effects. Experience has helped doctors find ways to manage and treat the adverse effects of drugs so that patients can tolerate their treatment better.

and bladder cancers, in combination with other cancer drugs. It causes severe effects on the nerves and the kidneys as well as severe nausea and vomiting during therapy, requiring very careful dosing and monitoring of patients who take it. Cisplatin's effect on the nerves can cause deafness to develop. Cisplatin is such an effective anticancer agent, however, that carboplatin, another platinum-containing molecule, was created in an attempt to improve on the toxicity problems. Carboplatin is not only less toxic than cisplatin at effective doses, but offers more predictable dosing. It can replace cisplatin in many of its uses, and is approved for the treatment of ovarian cancer. Its major adverse effect is myelosuppression. Carboplatin causes some of the same toxic reactions that cisplatin does, but less severely and less frequently.

Oxaliplatin is the newest member of this group of alkylating agents. It is approved for the treatment of cancers of the colon and rectum. It is less toxic to the kidneys than cisplatin, and it affects the nerves differently. Oxaliplatin does not alter hearing as cisplatin can, but it causes numbness, discomfort, and pain that can take many months to go away. In addition, it can cause prickling, blistering, and peeling of the palms of the hands and the soles of the feet, a collection of symptoms known as **hand-foot syndrome.**

ADVERSE EFFECTS OF ALKYLATING AGENTS

Nitrogen mustard gas was useful as a chemical warfare agent because of its extremely irritating effect on human tissues. Victims of exposure experienced painful blistering and peeling of their skin and mucous membranes. Administered as an anticancer treatment, alkylating agents are manufactured for safe administration usually as intravenous injections or as tablets to be taken orally. Even so, local irritation and injury at the site of injection is common with some of these drugs. Alkylating agents can also cause myelosuppression. This can pose a problem for patients, especially if they are not being treated for leukemia or lymphoma. A lack of normal bone marrow function can lead to **immunosuppression** (weakened immune system function) and an increased risk of infection. **Alopecia** (hair loss) and **anorexia** (prolonged loss of appetite) are also common adverse effects with the use of alkylating agents.

3

Antimetabolites

Around the time that scientists were first working on using the nitrogen mustards to "poison" cancer cells, a pathologist at Children's Hospital in Boston tried a different strategy to eliminate cancer. In the mid-1940s, Dr. Sidney Farber noticed that children with leukemia who were given large doses of the vitamin folic acid to boost their red blood cell production suffered a rapid acceleration of their cancer. He concluded that blocking the action of folic acid in the body would stop the disease. Farber acquired several folic acid **antagonists** (agents that oppose the action of another chemical). A chemical called aminopterin, given to him by the drug company Lederle, improved the condition of 10 out of 16 seriously ill children with leukemia.

The report of Farber's findings in the prestigious *New England Journal of Medicine* excited a great deal of interest in his discovery. A local charitable group donated money to help Farber study this potential cure for leukemia further. The story of one of his patients, identified only as Jimmy, captured the sympathy of the nation and inspired many people to donate money to buy Jimmy a television set so he could watch his favorite team, the Boston Braves, play baseball.

Farber is remembered today for the work that led to the development of methotrexate, which is still used to treat leukemia; for creating the Children's Cancer Research Foundation, known today as the Dana-Farber Cancer Institute; and for inspiring the creation of the Jimmy Fund, which continues to raise money for cancer research in the 21st century.

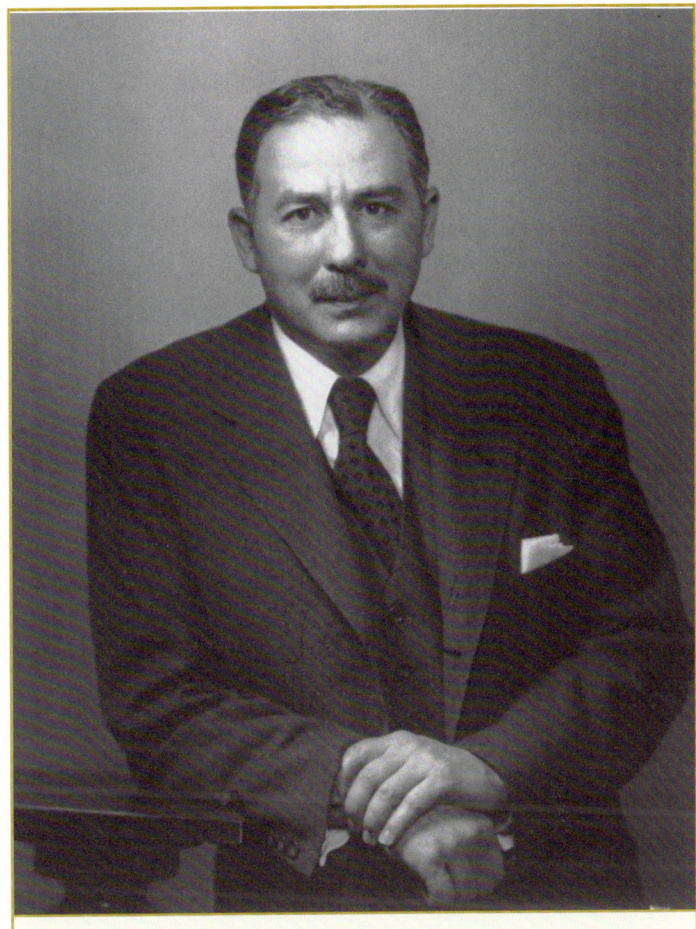

Figure 3.1 Dr. Sidney Farber. © National Library of Medicine

Since Farber's time, other researchers have discovered drugs that block different functions involved in cell growth and replication. Because they ultimately stop normal cellular metabolism, these drugs were called antimetabolites. This chapter discusses how these chemicals fool the cell into using these chemical look-alikes with deadly consequences for tumors.

ANTIMETABOLITE DRUGS

Table 3.1 lists the currently available antimetabolite cancer drugs in the United States. They are all **analogs** (chemical compounds that are structurally similar to, but slightly different from, another compound) of chemicals that are normally essential for cellular functions.

How Do Antimetabolites Work?

The antimetabolite drugs mimic compounds that cells normally need to carry out their functions, but they are just different enough that they stop these processes. Unable to carry out the processes necessary for life, the cells die. Understanding how these analogs work will require some knowledge about what DNA and RNA are made of.

In Chapter 1, we discussed the double-stranded structure of DNA. DNA provides a code from which cells get the information they need to manufacture all the proteins they need to sustain their activities. Antimetabolite drugs disrupt the stable DNA structure, making it impossible for the cell to continue the metabolic processes that keep it alive.

RNA is a single-stranded chain of molecules very similar to DNA. The string of the RNA strand is built from the sugar ribose instead of the deoxyribose used in DNA. Instead of the base thymine, RNA uses the base uracil. RNA is the molecule that the cell uses to decode the genes in DNA. Therefore, RNA is critical to the production of every protein created by a cell. Some of the antimetabolite drugs affect both RNA and DNA. RNA and DNA are referred to as nucleic acids, since they are both found in the nucleus of the cell.

Folic Acid Analogs, or Antifolates

Folic acid is an essential dietary nutrient for humans. Cells use folic acid to manufacture several critical molecules, including purines. The folic acid analogs methotrexate and pemetrexed specifically interfere with the normal use of folic acid by cells.

Table 3.1 Antimetabolic Drugs in the United States

Many of these agents are also available in generic form through various manufacturers.		
Category	Generic name (alternative name)	Trademark name (manufacturer or distributor)
Folic acid analogs	Methotrexate sodium	(generic; produced by various manufacturers)
	Pemetrexed	Alimta® (Eli Lilly and Company)
Pyrimidine analogs	Fluorouracil (5-fluorouracil, 5-FU)	(generic; produced by various manufacturers)
	Floxuridine (fluorodeoxyuridine)	FUDR® (Roche)
	Cytarabine (cytosine arabinoside)	(generic; produced by various manufacturers)
	Capecitabine	Xeloda® (Roche)
	Gemcitabine	Gemzar® (Eli Lilly and Company)
Purine analogs and related inhibitors	Mercaptopurine (6-mercaptopurine, 6-MP)	Purinethol® (GlaxoSmithKline) (also generic; produced by variou manufacturers)
	Thioguanine	(generic; GlaxoSmithKline)
	Pentostatin	Nipent® (SuperGen)
	Cladribine	Leustatin® (Ortho Biotech)
	Fludarabine	Fludara® (Berlex Laboratories)

As with all anticancer drugs, normal cells are affected, too, but they are usually better able to recover from the drug's effects than cancer cells are.

In a normal cell, an enzyme converts folic acid to a form that the cell can use as it makes the purines it needs. Antifolates fool cancer cells in two important ways:

• Cells that try to take up folic acid from their environment incorporate the antifolate instead;

• Once inside, the cell tries to use the antifolate the same way it normally uses folic acid, but is unable to change the

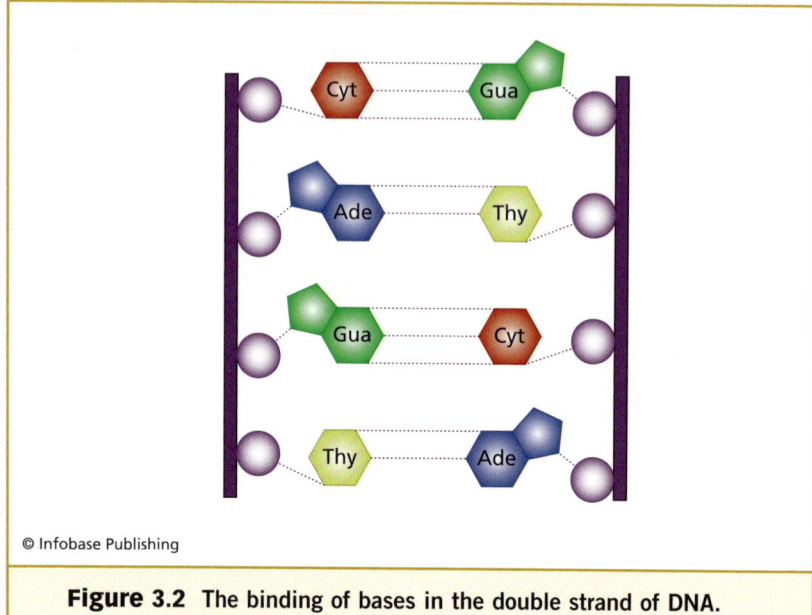

Figure 3.2 The binding of bases in the double strand of DNA.

antifolate drug the same way, ultimately depriving the cell of purines—crucial DNA building blocks.

Cells constantly and rapidly divide and grow in developing embryos. The embryo needs folic acid from the mother's circulation to adequately produce purines for all the new DNA it is manufacturing. This is why folic acid analogs given to a pregnant woman are toxic to the embryo and can cause miscarriage if taken during pregnancy.

Methotrexate is used for the treatment of gestational choriocarcinoma, chorioadenoma destruens, and hydatidiform mole. These are cancers arising from abnormal fertilization and growth of an embryo.

Methotrexate can be used alone or in combination with other anticancer agents to treat breast cancer, squamous cell cancers of the head and neck, advanced mycosis fungoides (a type of lymphoma), and lung cancer, particularly squamous cell and small cell types. Methotrexate is also used with other chemotherapeutic agents in the treatment of advanced-stage non-Hodgkin's lymphomas. It is also approved for treating some noncancerous diseases such as psoriasis and certain types of arthritis, and may be given orally or intravenously.

Pemetrexed is used, in combination with cisplatin, for the treatment of malignant pleural mesothelioma. This is a rare cancer of the cells of a membrane (**pleura**) that lines the abdominal cavity, heart, and lungs, and often occurs in response to asbestos exposure. Pemetrexed is also used as a single-agent therapy for non-small cell lung cancer (NSCLC).

Pemetrexed is given by intravenous infusion only. Patients also receive folic acid and vitamin B_{12} supplements during therapy to help their normal cells recover from toxicities.

LUNG CANCER CELLS

Most organs of the body are made up of more than one kind of cell, and the lungs are no exception. When doctors want to precisely describe a lung cancer, they try to determine what kind of lung cell the cancer arose from.

The majority of lung cancer cells fall into to two broad categories: Small-cell and Non-small cell (NSCLC). About 20 percent of lung cancers are small-cell cancers, and there are three subtypes of small-cell cancer: Small-cell carcinoma (also called oat cell cancer), mixed small cell/large cell carcinoma, and combined small cell carcinoma. Non-small cell cancer accounts for about 80 percent of lung cancer and there are nine subtypes. The majority of NSCLC cancers fall into three of these subtypes: Squamous cell carcinoma, large cell carcinoma, and adenocarcinoma. There are some other types of tissue in the lung, but these rarely become cancerous, and account for only a small percentage of lung cancers.

Pyrimidine Analogs

The pyrimidine analogs—which include fluorouracil (5-FU), floxuridine, cytarabine, capecitabine, and gemcitabine—share the ability to either block the cell's production of pyrimidines, or be successfully incorporated into the cell's DNA or RNA. They interfere with the resulting DNA's or RNA's ability to function normally. Some of these drugs can do both.

Floxuridine and capecitabine are metabolized by the liver, which turns them into 5-FU. Their anticancer activities are caused by the 5-FU that is produced. The cell incorporates 5-FU into both RNA and DNA. As a result, cell growth is impaired. Cells that are actively growing incorporate these drugs more readily, so tumor cells and the frequently dividing cells of the body (such as those in the bone marrow, gastrointestinal tract, hair follicles, and nails) are most affected. The activity of 5-FU is enhanced by a chemical called leucovorin, and patients often receive these drugs in combination.

5-FU is given by intravenous injection to treat cancer of the colon, rectum, breast, stomach, and pancreas. The FDA has not approved a tablet form of the drug, which is in common use in other countries. Floxuridine is given by **intraarterial** (into the artery) injection into the liver to treat gastrointestinal tumors that have spread to the liver. Capecitabine is an oral drug that is used in combination therapy to treat advanced and **metastatic** (cancer that has spread to a site in the body that is distant from where it originated) colon and breast cancers. Diarrhea can be a serious problem for patients who take this drug.

Gemcitabine both inhibits the cell enzymes that create the pyrimidine bases and replaces cytosine in the manufacture of DNA, effectively stopping the production of any DNA strand into which it is incorporated. It is used in combination therapy for advanced or metastatic breast and non–small cell lung cancers and as a single agent treatment for advanced or metastatic pancreatic cancer.

Once it is metabolized in the liver, cytarabine, like gemcitabine, inhibits DNA synthesis and gets incorporated into DNA. Also like gemcitabine, it is effective because it stops the manufacture of DNA so that the cell cannot grow and divide. It can be given by intravenous infusion or injection, **subcutaneously** (under the skin) or **intrathecally** (into the spinal fluid). Cytarabine is approved for use in combination therapy for the treatment of certain kinds of leukemia. In addition to the expected reactions to drugs of this class, cytarabine may cause a collection of symptoms called cytarabine syndrome, which can include fever, muscle aches, bone pain, chest pain, and rash. These problems can be treated with corticosteroids, which are potent **anti-inflammatory** drugs.

Purine Analogs and Related Inhibitor

Purine analogs and their related inhibitors include mercaptopurine, thioguanine, pentostatin, cladribine, and fludarabine. Mercaptopurine and thioguanine become analogs of guanine after they are metabolized in the body. Pentostatin is an analog of adenosine, and blocks an enzyme that normally processes adenosine. These agents strongly inhibit enzymes that are needed to synthesize DNA and RNA and may even be incorporated into their strands. As a result, they sabotage the production of both the nucleic acids and protein building blocks of cell replication.

Mercaptopurine is an oral drug approved for use alone and in combination therapy for certain types of leukemia. In addition to the expected bone marrow suppression, this drug may cause liver toxicity.

Thioguanine is close in chemical structure to mercaptopurine. It is also given orally. It is approved for use in combination therapy for nonlymphocytic leukemia.

CAN CANCER CELLS RESIST THERAPY?

Cancer cells can resist therapy. When this happens, a tumor that originally responded to therapy may start to grow again.

Resistance is not fully understood, but it may result from a kind of selective breeding. In Chapter 1, cancer cells were described as being able to keep dividing even when their DNA is damaged. Because these cells cannot repair their DNA, scientists think that a tumor is made up of a lot of mutant cells. Some of these mutations make the cells able to survive the activity of the drugs that are sent to kill it. Whether this means the cells simply make more of the enzyme or protein that the drug is inhibiting, or they create proteins that block the drugs, the mutants survive to replicate. When the survivors replicate, they are likely to pass on their special survival ability, and the tumor gradually becomes resistant. This is why combination regimens of chemotherapy are often used, to try to hit cancer cells in several different ways. If cancer cells become resistant to one drug in the regimen, they might still be vulnerable to the others.

Two possible mechanisms of drug resistance have already been mentioned: making more of the enzyme or protein that the cancer drug blocks and making proteins that block or deactivate the drug. There are other ways that cancer cells compensate for or evade the action of a drug, but one mechanism that can make the cell resistant to several drugs at once is the development of a multidrug resistance protein. These proteins act like a pump, moving potentially deadly drugs out of the cell. Research is ongoing into ways to reverse this defensive mechanism.

Pentostatin is used as a single-agent treatment for hairy-cell leukemia. Hairy-cell leukemia is an uncommon type of leukemia, accounting for less than 2 percent of all leukemias. The white blood cells in this cancer look fuzzy, or hairy, when viewed under the microscope. Rashes are common with this intravenous drug.

The metabolized products of cladribine and fludarabine interfere with DNA synthesis. In the case of cladribine, they are also incorporated into the DNA strands. Cladribine is unique in that it is toxic both to actively dividing cells and to nondividing living cells. Fludarabine is indicated for the treatment of B-cell chronic lymphocytic leukemia in patients whose disease progresses after other treatment. Cladribine is approved for the treatment of hairy-cell leukemia. Both are injectable drugs.

Adverse Effects of Antimetabolites

Antimetabolites commonly affect the rapidly dividing cells of the bone marrow and the **gastrointestinal system** (stomach and intestines), resulting in **mucositis**, bone marrow suppression, and thrombocytopenia (decreased blood levels of platelets, the cells responsible for blood clotting). These problems usually clear up soon after dosing is stopped. Methotrexate can sometimes cause an inflammation of the lung called pneumonitis, which also clears up rapidly when the drug is discontinued. In patients who also suffer from psoriasis or rheumatoid arthritis, antimetabolites may cause **cirrhosis** (disrupted structure and function) of the liver. Folic acid analogs can harm developing embryos and should not be given to pregnant women. Pregnancy should also be avoided in patients who are taking these drugs.

4

Natural Products

Ancient Egyptian physicians may have recognized cancer as early as 3000 B.C.E. Hieroglyphic inscriptions and papyri they left behind not only describe **benign** (harmless) and malignant (cancerous) tumors but also list a number of animal and plant mixtures that they used in an attempt to treat cancer. Although they removed some tumors surgically, they also recorded using barley compounds, pigs' ears, castor oil, and other natural substances to treat cancers of the stomach and uterus. The results of these treatments are unknown.

Later physicians observed that cancer usually returned after it was removed by surgery. In the first century C.E., Roman physician Celsus wrote, "After **excision**, even when a scar has formed, nonetheless the disease has returned." In the second century, Roman doctor Galen recorded his extensive medical observations. His views set the pattern of medical thought for nearly 1,000 years. Since he considered cancer an incurable disease that was resistant even to surgical removal, there seemed to be little hope for successful treatment of this disease through most of medical history. As a result, effective treatments for cancer were slow to develop.

Despite these barriers to treatment, people continued to turn to the natural world to try to cure cancer, much as the Egyptians had done. Historians have found records of many plant substances used to treat tumors. Some examples include:

- castor plant (*Ricinus communis*; produces castor oil)

- squirting cucumber (*Ecballium elaterium*; a common plant in the Mediterranean historically used as a strong laxative)

- deadly nightshade, also called belladonna (*Atropa belladonna*; several drugs are made from this plant)

- myrrh, which is the dried sap of the *Commiphora myrrha* tree

- frankincense, which is the dried sap of the *Boswellia thurifera* tree

- nettle, a plant in the genus Urtica; stinging nettle (*Urtica dioica*) is a common weed in Europe, Asia and North America.

Modern scientists investigated many of these ancient natural cures, and many were actually found to have anticancer activity. This chapter discusses the cancer drugs of natural origin that are in use today.

VINCA ALKALOIDS

The vinca alkaloids, which include vinblastine, vincristine, and vinorelbine, are a related group of molecules derived from the periwinkle plant *Catharanthus roseus*. This plant grows in warm climates, including the southern United States, and has a long history of medicinal use all over the world. While studying its possible use for treating diabetes in 1958, scientists discovered that an extract of periwinkle suppressed bone marrow production of blood cells. This led to an exploration of its activity against cancer.

How the Vinca Alkaloids Work

All vinca alkaloids work in a cell-cycle specific manner, stopping mitosis and causing cell death. In Chapter 1, mitosis was described as the phase in the cell cycle (M phase) when the cell finishes duplicating its genetic material and divides its contents and DNA into two cells. Figure 4.4 shows how the cell carefully lines up its chromosomes (tightly coiled molecules of DNA found in the nucleus of a cell) alongside fibers called

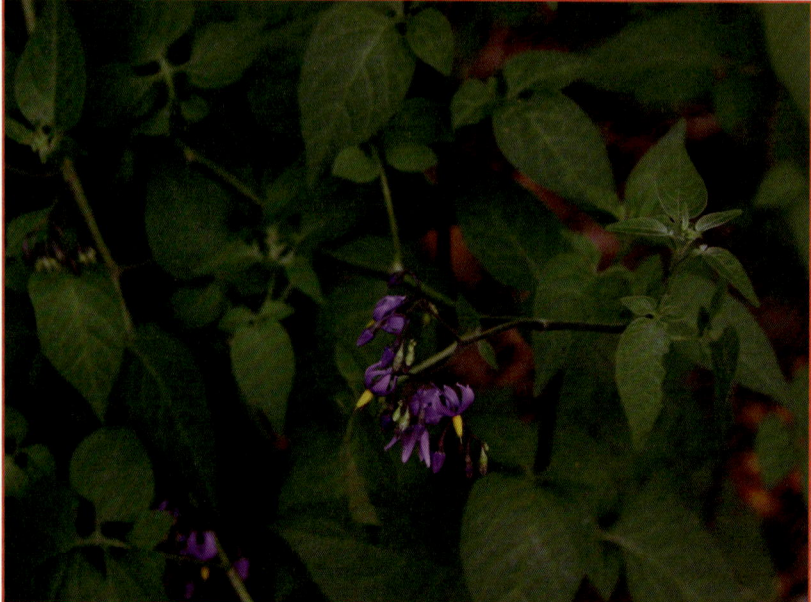

Figure 4.1 Deadly nightshade. Other plants in the same family as the deadly nightshade are not as toxic: tomato, potato, pepper, and eggplant. © Sue Sweeney/TheMondayGarden.com

microtubules. The vinca alkaloids interfere with the formation of these microtubules. Without them, the cell cannot divide and eventually dies.

Uses and Characteristics of the Vinca Alkaloids

Although chemically similar, these agents have unique and specific antitumor activities. Vincristine is a standard part of regimens used to treat pediatric leukemias and solid tumors, and is often used to treat adult lymphomas. Vinblastine is used mainly to treat lymphomas, cancer of the testicles, and advanced solid tumors of certain types. Although all the vinca alkaloids have adverse effects on the nervous system, vinblastine is less likely to be neurotoxic which makes it easier to use

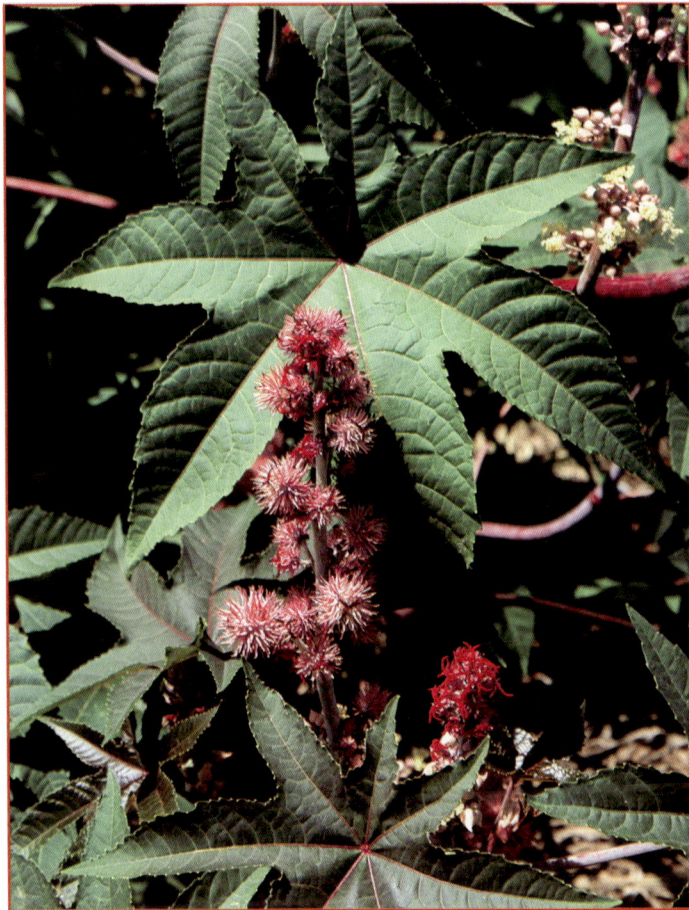

Figure 4.2 Castor bean plant. Castor oil is derived from the beans of this plant. The beans are also a source of the highly toxic substance, ricin. © Michael P. Gadomski/Photo Researchers, Inc.

safely in combination treatments. Vinorelbine is active against non-small cell lung cancer and breast cancer.

Adverse Effects of the Vinca Alkaloids

Myelosuppression can occur within a week to ten days after a patient takes vinblastine or vinorelbine, but vincristine generally causes little effect on blood cell production. All three drugs cause hair loss. All three drugs also can cause numbness and tingling in the hands and feet due to nerve damage (neuro-toxicity), but this effect is most predictable for vincristine. The numbness and tingling can progress to muscle weakness. High-dose therapies of vincristine can result in severe constipation.

TAXANES (MICROTUBULE POLYMER STABILIZERS)

The microtubule polymer stabilizers, or taxanes, include doc-etaxel and paclitaxel. The first taxane, paclitaxel, was extracted from the bark of the slow-growing Pacific yew tree. Harvesting the bark kills the tree, making this an expensive and ecologi-cally damaging way to produce the drug, so better methods were developed. Luckily, a closely related chemical compound could be easily extracted from the leaves of an easily renewable

NATURAL MEDICINES IN THE MODERN WORLD

Between the years 40 and 90 c.e., a Greek physician named Dioscorides wrote a five-volume collection called *De Materia Medica*, describing the medicinal substances in use at that time. About 80 percent of the substances he mentioned were plant-derived medicines. The rest came from minerals and animals. In 1976, a report described the sources of medicines in current use, and the comparison to *De Materia Medica* is interesting. Keep in mind that many modern drugs in the 1970s came from plants. Without accounting for all drug sources, the approximate proportions were: 50 percent were synthetic, 25 percent were from plants, 7 percent were from minerals, and 6 percent were from animals. Later reports stated that 62 percent of the anticancer drugs available in the United States before 1983 could be related to natural sources.

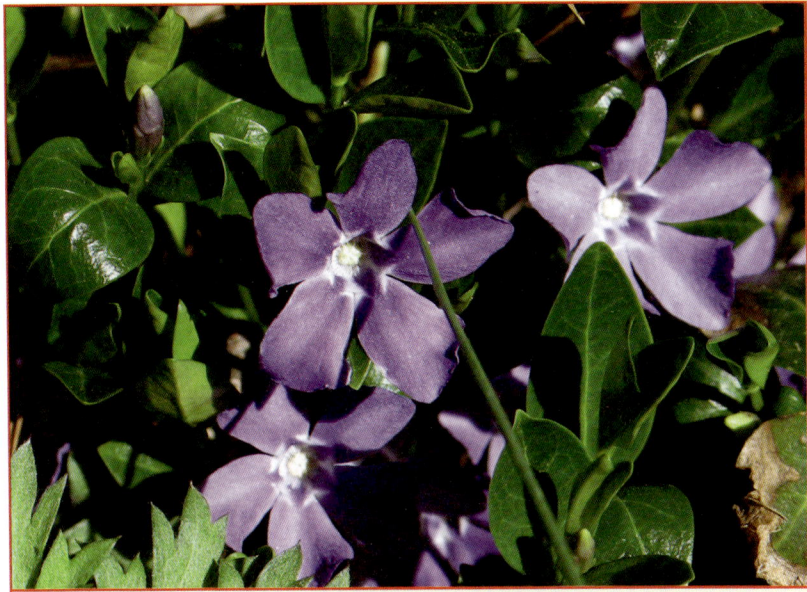

Figure 4.3 The vinca plant; also called dogbane. © Sue Sweeney/TheMondayGarden.com

source, the ornamental shrub *Taxus baccata*. The compound extracted from the leaves is chemically transformed to make paclitaxel.

How Taxanes Work

Like the vinca alkaloids, the taxanes stop mitosis, but instead of inhibiting microtubule formation, the taxanes promote it. However, they also bind the microtubules into bundles and abnormal shapes, which keeps the tubules from performing the important function of organizing cell contents during division.

Uses and Characteristics of the Microtubule Polymer Stabilizers

Both paclitaxel and docetaxel are used in the treatment of advanced breast cancer and non-small cell lung cancers.

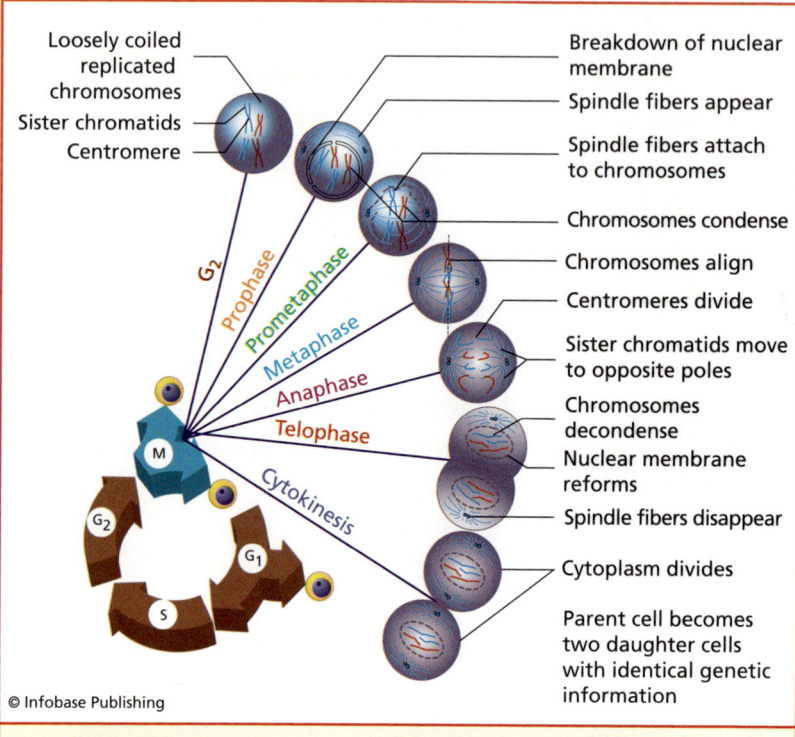

Loosely coiled replicated chromosomes
Sister chromatids
Centromere

Breakdown of nuclear membrane
Spindle fibers appear
Spindle fibers attach to chromosomes
Chromosomes condense
Chromosomes align
Centromeres divide
Sister chromatids move to opposite poles
Chromosomes decondense
Nuclear membrane reforms
Spindle fibers disappear
Cytoplasm divides
Parent cell becomes two daughter cells with identical genetic information

G₂
Prophase
Prometaphase
Metaphase
Anaphase
Telophase
Cytokinesis
M
G₂
G₁
S

© Infobase Publishing

Figure 4.4 The cell cycle and movement of chromosomes, guided by microtubules.

Paclitaxel is also used to treat advanced ovarian cancer. Docetaxel is used to treat advanced prostate cancer that does not depend on the hormone androgen to grow. Prostate cancer that depends on androgen to grow is better treated with other agents that will be described in Chapter 5, Hormones and Hormone Antagonists.

Adverse Effects of Microtubule Polymer Stabilizers

The taxanes suppress bone marrow function, and, in high-dose regimens, can cause **neuropathy** and **mucositis**. Paclitaxel is also associated with allergic reactions in some people, which can be severe enough to be fatal if the allergy is not recognized quickly. Patients who take paclitaxel are pretreated with

Table 4.1 Vinka Alkaloids Available in the United States

Generic Name	Trademarked name (manufacturer or distributor)
Vinblastine	Velban® (Eli Lilly)
Vincristine	Oncovin® (Eli Lilly)
Vinorelbine	Navelbine® (GlaxoSmithKline)

antihistamines and steroid drugs to avoid serious allergy symptoms. Docetaxel is more likely to cause fluid retention that could lead to breathing problems and heart (**cardiac**) rhythm abnormalities. Premedicating the patient with steroids can help avoid these complications.

ANTIBIOTIC ANTICANCER AGENTS

Antibiotic anticancer agents include dactinomycin, daunorubicin, doxorubicin, epirubicin, idarubicin, valrubicin, mitoxantrone, bleomycin, and mitomycin. As the name of this class of drugs suggests, these anticancer drugs are all related to antibiotics, drugs commonly used to treat bacterial infections. The early precursors of the antibiotics were chemical compounds first found in bacteria grown in the laboratory. Most of the antibiotics in use today are chemically modified forms of the agents first extracted from bacterial cultures.

The antibiotic anticancer agents were all isolated from different species of the fungus *Streptomyces*. Actinomycin A was

Table 4.2 The Taxanes

Generic Name	Trademarked name (manufacturer or distributor)
Paclitaxel	Taxol® (Bristol-Myers Squibb)
Docetaxel	Taxotere® (Sanofi Aventis)

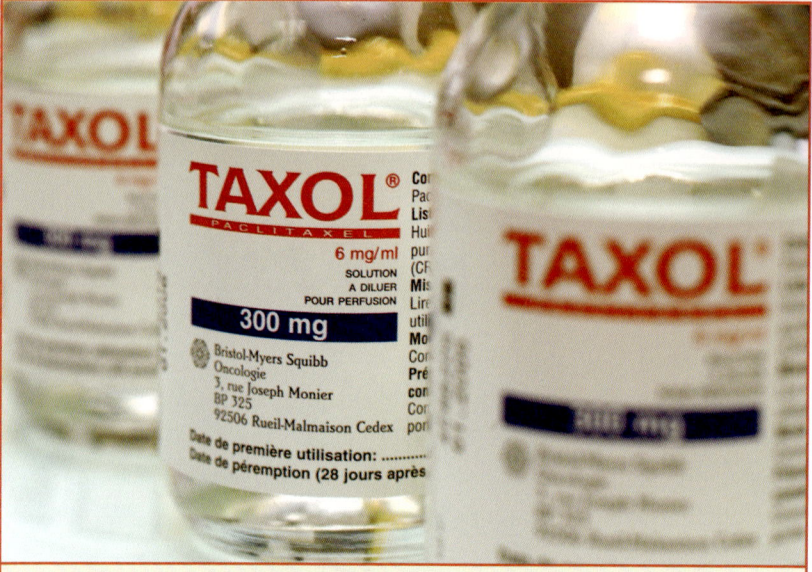

Figure 4.5 Taxol, a derivative of the pacific Yew tree used in chemotherapy. © Alix/Phanie/Photo Researchers, Inc.

the first antibiotic extracted. Actinomycin D, or dactinomycin, proved to have anticancer effects. Daunorubicin, doxorubicin, epirubicin, idarubicin, valrubicin, and mitoxantrone are related by a basic chemical structure they share with the well-known antibiotic tetracycline. This structure gives this group the name *anthracyclines*. Although isolated from different strains of *Streptomyces*, bleomycin and mitomycin share a structure that makes them active against some difficult-to-treat cancers, and gives them toxicities that favor their use in potent combination treatments.

How the Antibiotic Anticancer Agents Work

Dactinomycin binds to the double strand of DNA. This keeps the strands from separating the way they normally would as they prepare for having their genetic code decoded by RNA, a

Table 4.3 The Antibiotic Anticancer Agents

Generic Name	Trademarked name (manufacturer or distributor)
Dactinomycin	Cosmegen® (Merck)
Daunorubicin	Cerubidine® (Bedford Labs)
Doxorubicin	Adriamycin® (Adria Laboratories)
	Rubex® (Bristol-Myers Squibb)
Doxorubicin, liposomal	Doxil® (Ortho Biotech)
Epirubicin	Ellence® (Pfizer)
Idarubicin	Idamycin® (Adria Laboratories)
Valrubicin	Valstar® (Anthra Pharmaceuticals; Medeva Pharmaceuticals)
Mitoxantrone	Novantrone® (Serono Pharmaceuticals)
Bleomycin	Blenoxane® (Bristol-Myers Squibb)
Mitomycin	Mutamycin® (Bristol-Myers Squibb)

process called **transcription**, and replication. If the DNA cannot be transcribed, the cell cannot divide. This makes dactinomycin a potent antitumor agent, since it stops the rapid cell division of cancers.

The anthracyclines (daunorubicin, doxorubicin, epirubicin, idarubicin, valrubicin, and mitoxantrone) affect DNA in multiple ways. They directly alter the DNA strands, affect the molecules involved in the creation of DNA and its proteins, and cause oxygen in the cell to chemically react with DNA, damaging it. Cells damaged this way become unable to follow through with the process of cell division, and so they die.

Mitomycin is metabolized by cellular enzymes, turning into a chemical that acts like the alkylating agents do (see Chapter 2). It cross-links the DNA strands, inhibiting its ability to replicate when the cell is ready to divide.

Uses and Characteristics of the Antibiotic Anticancer Agents

Dactinomycin is most important in the treatment of two tumors that usually occur in children: rhabdomyosarcoma (a tumor arising from muscle tissue) and Wilm's tumor (a kidney tumor). It is commonly used in combination with radiation and other agents to treat these diseases. Dactinomycin is also useful for the treatment of Ewing's sarcoma and gestational trophoblastic tumors (tumors that arise from tissues in the uterus that normally support the growth of a fetus).

Daunorubicin is used to treat AIDS-related Kaposi's sarcoma, and is useful in the treatment of certain leukemias, particularly acute lymphocytic leukemia (ALL) and acute myelogenous leukemia (AML).

Doxorubicin is effective for many leukemias and lymphomas, but is also active against a number of solid tumors, especially breast cancer, ovarian cancer, and small-cell cancer of the lung. To increase a cancer's exposure to this drug, a special formulation of doxorubucin called liposomal doxorubicin is available. When the drug molecules are enclosed in a fatty coating called a **liposome**, the doxorubicin stays in the patient's bloodstream longer. Liposomal doxorubicin is an injectable drug that is most often used to treat ovarian cancer and Kaposi's sarcoma.

Epirubuicin is primarily used to treat cancers of the breast, esophagus, lung, ovary, and stomach; Hodgkin's and non-Hodgkin's lymphoma; and soft tissue sarcomas. Idarubicin is useful in treating certain leukemias.

Valrubicin is used exclusively in the treatment of bladder cancer. It is administered directly into the bladder through a thin tube (**catheter**) once a week for six weeks. The most common side effects of this treatment are bladder irritation, a strong urge to urinate, and frequent urination.

Mitoxantrone is used to treat acute nonlymphocytic leukemia, breast and ovarian cancers, and non-Hodgkin's and Hodgkin's lymphomas. In addition to its more serious adverse effects, listed earlier in this chapter, mitoxantrone can temporarily turn the urine blue or green.

Bleomycin is used in the treatment of many different cancers, including cancers of the testes, head and neck, penis, cervix, vulva, anus, and skin. It is also active in Hodgkin's and non-Hodgkin's lymphomas and helps stop the accumulation of fluid in the membranes surrounding the lung (**pleural effusions**). This drug may be given by intravenous or intramuscular injection.

Mitomycin is dosed intravenously in the treatment of esophagus, stomach, anal, and pancreas cancers. Like valrubicin, it can be administered directly into the bladder to treat bladder cancers.

Adverse Effects of the Antibiotic Anticancer Agents

Dactinomycin typically causes nausea and vomiting within a few hours after dosing. Bone marrow suppression may occur within a week after completing therapy. Inflammation and ulceration of the mucous membranes of the mouth, and diarrhea are also common.

The anthracyclines (daunorubicin, doxorubicin, epirubicin, idarubicin, valrubicin, and mitoxantrone) typically cause myelosuppression, which can become severe enough to limit the dose of these drugs. Inflammation of the mouth, gastrointestinal problems, and hair loss are common, but can be reversed after dosing stops. These drugs may also affect the heart muscle, causing short-term (**acute**) and long-term (chronic) changes. The acute effects include changes in the way the heart beats (**arrhythmias**) and even heart failure, when the heart becomes unable to pump enough blood through the body. The chronic changes accumulate over time, resulting in congestive heart failure that resists the usual treatments. The risk of heart failure occurring is minimized by keeping the doses low and by using drugs that protect the heart (**cardioprotective**) at the same time. Most of the anthracyclines also cause the urine to harmlessly and temporarily turn red. This is not from blood, but from the color of the drugs and their metabolites. The anthracyclines are all given intravenously, usually by slow infusion, because they can be irritating, especially if they leak outside of the vein into the local tissues (**extravasation**).

Bleomycin and mitomycin have very different toxicities. Bleomycin causes skin effects, including redness, ulceration, and overproduction of pigment (**hyperpigmentation**) that leaves dark spots, especially where ulceration occurred. Bleomycin also causes lung (**pulmonary**) toxicity. This can start with a dry cough, then lead to the collection of fluid in the lung, and may even progress to life-threatening scar tissue formation (**fibrosis**) in the lungs. The risk of pulmonary toxicity increases at high doses and in patients over 70 years of age. Because bleomycin does not cause myelosupression, there is a significant advantage to using it in combination with other anticancer drugs.

Mitomycin's major toxic effect is myelosuppression. In high doses, it may cause pulmonary fibrosis. In combination therapy with doxorubicin, it can make the cardiac toxicity of doxorubicin worse.

TOPOISOMERASE INHIBITORS

The topoisomersase inhibitors—irinotecan, topotecan, etoposide phosphate, and teniposide—share a mechanism of action, but are divided by their sources. Camptothecin was isolated in 1966 from a Chinese tree, *Camptotheca acuminata*, and demonstrated anticancer properties. Camptothecin proved too toxic for use in people, but safer and more stable compounds were developed throughout the 1980s, leading to the creation of irinotecan and topotecan. Teniposide and etoposide both come from a chemical extracted from the mandrake plant, or mayapple, which was used as a folk remedy by Native Americans and early American colonists.

How Topoisomerase Inhibitors Work

During cell division, the double-stranded DNA in the nucleus must unwind, split apart temporarily while its two halves get copied, then reattach and rewind. Topoisomerase enzymes aid this process by causing small, deliberate breaks in the strands that relieve the stress of untwisting. After the strands are replicated, topoisomerases repair the breaks as the strands twist back together. Inhibitors of this enzyme interfere with the cell's ability to repair the breaks and reconstruct the double-stranded helix of DNA. As a result, the cell cannot finish dividing, and dies. These drugs act only on cells that are in the appropriate phase of their life cycle.

Uses and Characteristics of the Topoisomerase Inhibitors

Irinotecan is used as a component of **first-line therapy** (the first attempt to treat a newly diagnosed patient's cancer) in combination with 5-fluorouracil and leucovorin for patients with metastatic carcinoma of the colon or rectum. Irinotecan is also indicated for patients with metastatic carcinoma of the colon or rectum whose disease has recurred or progressed following initial fluorouracil-based therapy. It is available as an intravenous injection.

Topotecan is approved for the treatment of two kinds of cancer, by intravenous injection:

- metastatic carcinoma of the ovary after failure of prior chemotherapy;

- a particular type of small-cell lung cancer after first-line chemotherapy fails.

Etoposide is available as an intravenous injection and as capsules. In either form, it is indicated for treating two different cancers:

- **Refractory** testicular tumors, in combination with other approved chemotherapeutic agents, in patients who have already received appropriate surgical, chemotherapeutic, and radiation therapy;

- Small-cell lung cancer, in combination with other approved chemotherapeutic agents, as first-line treatment.

Teniposide is approved for use in combination with other approved anticancer agents for **induction therapy** (therapy whose goal is to start reducing the size of the cancerous tumor in preparation for further treatment), in patients with refractory (resistant to treatment) childhood acute lymphoblastic leukemia (ALL). The goal of induction therapy is to minimize the cancer and evaluate its response to therapy before following up with treatment designed to eliminate any remaining disease.

Table 4.4 The Topoisomerase Inhibitors

Generic Name	Trademarked name (manufacturer or distributor)
Irinotecan	Camptosar® (Pfizer)
Topotecan	Hycamtin® (GlaxoSmithKline)
Etoposide phosphate	Etopophos®; Vepesid® (Bristol-Myers Squibb)
Teniposide	Vumon® (Bristol-Myers Squibb)

Adverse Effects

Bone marrow suppression, with its associated increased risk of infection and bleeding, is caused by all the topoisomerase inhibitors. Many of these agents also cause allergic reactions that can become life-threatening. More typically, they cause nausea, vomiting, weight loss, diarrhea, constipation, mucositis, headache, fever, muscle aches and pains, and alopecia.

All of the drugs in this class cause neutropenia (decreased levels of neutrophils, a type of white blood cell) and thrombocytopenia (reduced number of platelets in the blood). Nausea, vomiting, and diarrhea are also common.

Of this class of drugs, teniposide is most likely to cause a serious allergic reaction. Patients should be monitored closely for the sudden development of fever, chills, rash, hypotension, dyspnea (difficulty breathing), and changes in heart rhythm.

Irinotecan is more likely than the other agents in this class to produce serious diarrhea and inflammation of the intestinal tract.

5

Hormones and Hormone Antagonists

Hormones are chemicals that cells secrete into the bloodstream. They have an effect on some organ or other type of cell. The concept of hormones was first defined scientifically by Scottish physician Sir George Thomas Beatson. Beatson lived near sheep and cattle farms all his life, and probably knew about a typical practice of farmers at that time in which a cow's ovaries were removed shortly after it gave birth to a calf in order to keep the cow lactating (producing milk) indefinitely. In 1878, Beatson demonstrated changes in milk production in rabbits after he removed the ovaries, which suggested the idea of "one organ holding control over . . . another and separate organ" of the body. Specifically, he recognized that this information could hold promise for the treatment of breast cancer. When he tested his idea by removing the ovaries of advanced breast cancer patients, he often saw improvement. Beatson had discovered the role of the female hormone, estrogen, in breast cancer even before the existence of the hormone was known. His work ultimately led to the use of modern-day hormone therapies, which are discussed in detail in this chapter.

ANTICANCER HORMONE DRUGS

The body uses hormones to regulate many functions, including growth, digestion, sexual development, and reproduction, among others. Because of their diverse activity in the body, hormonally active drugs can have several therapeutic uses. In this chapter, only their anticancer activities will be discussed.

HOW THE HORMONES AND HORMONE ANTAGONISTS WORK

Many normal cells in the body grow and perform their regular functions in response to the presence of particular hormones. For example, the cells lining a woman's uterus proliferate in response to hormones released at the time of ovulation, and male testicular tissues produce sperm in response to the presence of hormones. Unfortunately, tumors sometimes arise from these hormone-sensitive cells. This can result in tumor tissue that grows vigorously in the presence of hormones and even depends on these hormones for its growth. Anticancer hormone therapy takes advantage of these characteristics by limiting, in different ways, the availability of hormones to the cells.

In both normal and cancer cells, hormones regulate which genes in the cell are stimulated to produce the cell's proteins and structures (see Figure 5.1).

EARLY SUCCESS WITH PROSTATE CANCER

Half a century after Beatson's discovery, Canadian-born American urologist Charles Huggins found during the 1930s that castration, or surgical removal of the testicles, of very advanced prostate cancer patients often brought rapid relief from the agony of their disease and could even prolong their lives. In 1966, he received the Nobel Prize in medicine for his discovery of the role male hormones play in prostate cancer, and for demonstrating that cancer that had spread widely throughout the body could be cured.

Table 5.1 Hormone and Hormone Antagonists

Generic Name	Trademarked name (manufacturer or distributor)
Tamoxifen	Nolvadex® (AstraZeneca)
Fulvestrant	Faslodex® (AstraZeneca)
Toremifene	Fareston® (Orion Corp.)
Medroxyprogesterone	Prempro® (Wyeth), Provera® (Pfizer); also generic by various manufacturers
Megestrol	Megace® (Bristol-Myers Squibb); also generic by various manufacturers
Anastrozole	Arimidex® (AstraZeneca)
Letrozole	Femara® (Novartis)
Exemestane	Aromasin® (Pfizer)
Goserelin	Zoladex® (AstraZeneca)
Leuprolide	Lupron® (TAP Pharmaceuticals), Eligard® (Sanofi Aventis); also generic by various manufacturers
Triptorelin	Trelstar® (Watson Pharma, Inc.)
Bicalutamide	Casodex® (AstraZeneca)
Flutamide	Eulexin® (Schering-Plough); also generic by various manufacturers
Nilutamide	Nilandron® (Sanofi Aventis)
Fluoxymesterone	Halotestin® (Pfizer); also generic by various manufacturers
Octreotide	Sandostatin® (Novartis); also generic by various manufacturers

Hormones are carried into the cell, where they interact with hormone receptors. In fact, tumor cells can be tested to determine which hormones they have receptors for. When the receptor connects with the right hormone, the receptor stimulates genes to produce proteins that go on to perform their

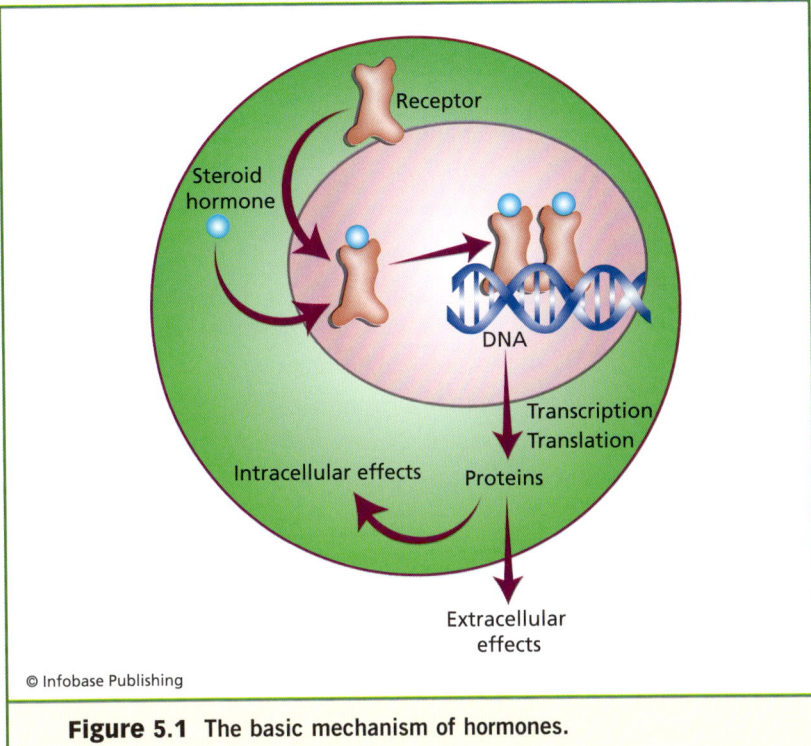

Figure 5.1 The basic mechanism of hormones.

© Infobase Publishing

functions in the cell. Interfering with hormones at any step along the way ultimately interferes with cell behavior. In the case of hormone-sensitive cancers that depend on the hormone for their uncontrolled growth, interference can end the life of the cancer. Groups of drugs in this category include selective estrogen receptor modulators (SERMS), progestins (megestrol acetate), luteinizing hormone-releasing hormone (LHRH) agonists, and androgenic agonists.

SELECTIVE ESTROGEN RECEPTOR MODULATORS (SERMS)

Estrogens and progestins are the major classes of steroidal female sex hormones. They are called steroidal because they share a basic chemical structure, known as sterol, which the body gets from converting cholesterol. The body manufactures estrogens and progestins in a process that first chemically converts cholesterol into male sex hormones, and then, step by step, into other steroids including the female sex hormones.

Both men and women produce both male and female sex hormones; men produce more of the male hormones, and women produce more of the female hormones. This is significant to the treatment of cancer, because both sexes are capable of developing tumors that respond to hormones that they are not producing in abundance. For example, men can and do develop estrogen-sensitive tumors.

The estrogen antagonists—tamoxifen, fulvestrant, toremifene, anastrozole, letrozole, and exemestane—are often referred to as selective estrogen receptor modulators (SERMs). This name reflects the fact that each SERM is more active in certain tissues than in others. One explanation for this is that there are two different estrogen receptors in the body. Alpha receptors are found mainly in the breast and uterus, and beta receptors are found in the bone and blood vessels. In addition, there are numerous compounds in the body that act in conjunction with estrogens (either at the

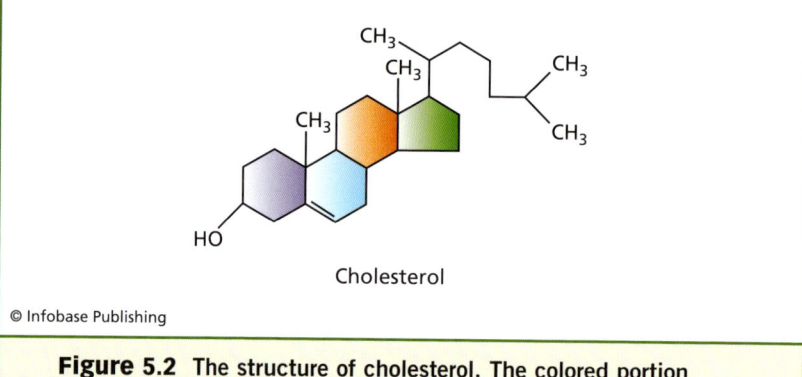

Cholesterol

© Infobase Publishing

Figure 5.2 The structure of cholesterol. The colored portion indicates the part of the molecule that these hormones all share, and that gives them the name, steroid.

receptors or at the genes) to slightly alter the ultimate cellular response to estrogens. Although it is not always clear which drug acts on which kind of receptor, it is clear that many drugs, particularly the newer agents, are relatively selective in their activity on tumor tissues. Their actions on nontumor tissues in the body account for many of their unwanted effects.

How SERMs Work

There are two broad categories of estrogen antagonists, defined by the way they work: antiestrogens and aromatase inhibitors. Table 5.2 lists the drugs by their mechanism of action.

The antiestrogens block cellular receptors for the steroidal female sex hormones. As you will see in the next section, the different antiestrogen drugs have slightly different effects on receptors, and are attracted to different types of cells in the body.

The aromatase inhibitors decrease the amount of estrogen produced in the body by inhibiting the enzyme aromatase. The body uses aromatase in the stepwise production of hormones from cholesterol. Aromatase makes the final conversion of male sex hormones into estrogens happen.

Uses and Characteristics of the SERMs

The SERMs mentioned here are all used to treat breast cancer, which is one cancer whose growth is typically stimulated by the

Table 5.2 The Antibiotic Anticancer Agents

Antiestrogens	Aromatase inhibitors
Tamoxifen	Anastrozole
Toremifene	Letrozole
Fulvestrant	Exemestane

presence of estrogens. About two-thirds of breast cancers contain receptors for estrogens. Breast cancer is rare in men. In fact, it is about 100 times more common in women, but when it occurs in a man, it is treated the same way it is treated in women, which includes the use of SERMs. These agents are currently being studied to better understand their long-term effects and to see how they compare with tamoxifen, which has the longest history and broadest use in breast cancer treatment. Each of the SERMs is available as a tablet. Their use in women can depend on whether the woman has experienced **menopause**, a time in life after which her body produces far less of the female sex hormones.

Adverse Effects and Characteristics of the SERMs

Tamoxifen was the first antiestrogen and is still in wide use today. Although it does block estrogen receptors and acts as an antagonist, it also has some estrogen-like activity, making it both an estrogen antagonist and a partial **agonist** (a drug that produces the same action as the substance it mimics). This has been a therapeutic advantage. Women run the risk of developing brittle, porous bones (**osteoporosis**) when they don't have enough estrogen. This is typical among women after menopause. If tamoxifen were too good at blocking this critical hormone, particularly in postmenopausal women, then patients on tamoxifen therapy would be at an even higher risk of developing osteoporosis, but this is not the case. In fact, tamoxifen therapy has beneficial effects on bone density and also on serum **lipid** (fat) levels. Unfortunately, tamoxifen use has also been linked to a slightly increased risk of both endometrial cancer (a cancer of the uterus) and **thromboembolic** (blockage of a blood vessel by a piece of a clot that breaks away) events. These risks occur most often in patients over the age of 50 and in those who take the drug for many years.

Each of the antiestrogens is being studied for its effect on bone density, serum lipids, blood clot formation, and cardiac

Table 5.3 The Approved Uses of the Estrogen Antagonists

Antiestrogens	Approved Uses
Tamoxifen	*Metastatic breast cancer*: Tamoxifen is effective in the treatment of metastatic breast cancer in both women and men. In premenopausal women with metastatic breast cancer, tamoxifen is an alternative to removal or destruction of the ovaries, an important source of hormone production in women.
	Adjuvant treatment of breast cancer: Following surgical removal of the breast (mastectomy) or radiation therapy, tamoxifen is used to treat post-menopausal women if some of the nearby lymph nodes had cancer cells in them and in some women without cancer cells in the lymph nodes.
	Reduction in breast cancer incidence in high-risk women: Tamoxifen is used to reduce the incidence of breast cancer in women who are at high risk for breast cancer or to decrease the risk of invasive cancer after treatment of local disease.
Toremifene	Toremifene is used to treat metastatic breast cancer in post-menopausal women with tumors whose cells have estrogen receptors (estrogen-positive) or tumors with unknown receptor status.
Fulvestrant	Fulvestrant is used to treat metastatic breast cancer in post-menopausal women whose tumor cells have sex hormone receptors, and who have failed treatment with antiestrogen therapy.
Aromatase inhibitors	
Anastrozole	Anastrozole is indicated for the treatment of advanced breast cancer in postmenopausal women whose disease worsens after tamoxifen therapy. Patients with tumors that have no estrogen receptors and patients who did not respond to previous tamoxifen therapy rarely benefit from treatment with anastrozole.
Letrozole	Letrozole is indicated for the extended adjuvant treatment of early breast cancer in postmenopausal women who have received five years of adjuvant tamoxifen therapy. It is also used for first-line treatment of postmenopausal women with locally advanced or metastatic breast cancer with tumors that have hormone receptors or for tumors whose hormone receptor status cannot be determined. Letrozole is also indicated for the treatment of advanced breast cancer in postmenopausal women whose disease progressed after antiestrogen therapy.
Exemestane	Exemestane is indicated for the treatment of advanced breast cancer in postmenopausal women whose disease has progressed following tamoxifen therapy.

(heart-related) health. Aside from these potential adverse effects, these drugs produce few other unwanted symptoms. On occasion, some nausea and gastrointestinal discomfort may occur early in therapy, as well some of the symptoms of menopause (hot flashes, menstrual irregularities, fatigue, water retention, and mood changes).

Toremifene is chemically similar to tamoxifen, but is not a steroid. Its long-term effects are still being studied. Like tamoxifen, it may have both estrogen antagonist and agonist characteristics. Raloxifene is also like tamoxifen in its beneficial effects on the bone. Fulvestrant not only blocks estrogen receptors, it also decreases the production of these receptors by the cells.

Aromatase inhibitors decrease the amount of circulating estrogen in the body, so the adverse events they cause are similar to the symptoms of menopause, which include hot flashes and occasional muscle weakness, fatigue, mood changes, joint and muscle aches and pains, nausea, and water retention. Osteoporosis and fractures are more common with the aromatase inhibitors than with tamoxifen. Anastrozole, letrozole, and exemestane share many characteristics and approved uses because of their specific action on the enzymes that convert male sex hormones (androgens) into estrogens.

PROGESTINS (MEGESTROL ACETATE)

The progestins are a group of chemicals that mimic the activity of a class of a hormone called progesterone. Progesterone plays an important role in maintaining the lining of the uterus during pregnancy, and in changing the breast tissues toward the end of pregnancy. It also has a variety of effects on metabolism.

The most common use of the progestins is in **contraceptives** (products that prevent pregnancy). Only one of these progestins, megestrol acetate, is also used to treat breast and endometrial (referring to the lining of the uterus) cancers. Megestrol acetate's precise mechanism of action against cancer is not well understood. It is known to be more effective in cancers whose cells have receptors for progesterone (progesterone-positive).

Uses and Characteristics of the Progestins

Megestrol acetate is indicated for the palliative treatment of advanced carcinoma of the breast or endometrium. **Advanced disease** is defined as recurrent, inoperable, or metastatic disease. Megestrol acetate often causes weight gain. Advanced disease patients typically lose a lot of weight, which can worsen their fatigue and weakness from their disease. There has been some research into using this drug to help cancer patients put on the weight they are losing. It is available as a tablet and a liquid for oral administration.

ANDROGEN ANTAGONISTS

Androgens are male steroidal hormones, produced in the body as part of the production of hormones from cholesterol. One example of an androgen is testosterone; testosterone and other androgens are almost exclusively produced in the testicles. The antiandrogen (androgen antagonist) drugs, including bicalutamide, flutamide, and nilutamide, powerfully block the activity of androgens on androgen receptors, so they are useful in treating androgen-sensitive tumors. Their blocking activity is so complete that their action is referred to as chemical castration. Their action is reversible. In other words, when a patient stops taking the drugs, the androgen blockade gradually goes away. This is clearly preferable to the permanent effects of surgical castration.

Uses and Characteristics of the Androgen Antagonists

These drugs are approved only to treat prostate cancer. Bicalutamide and flutamide are approved for combination therapy

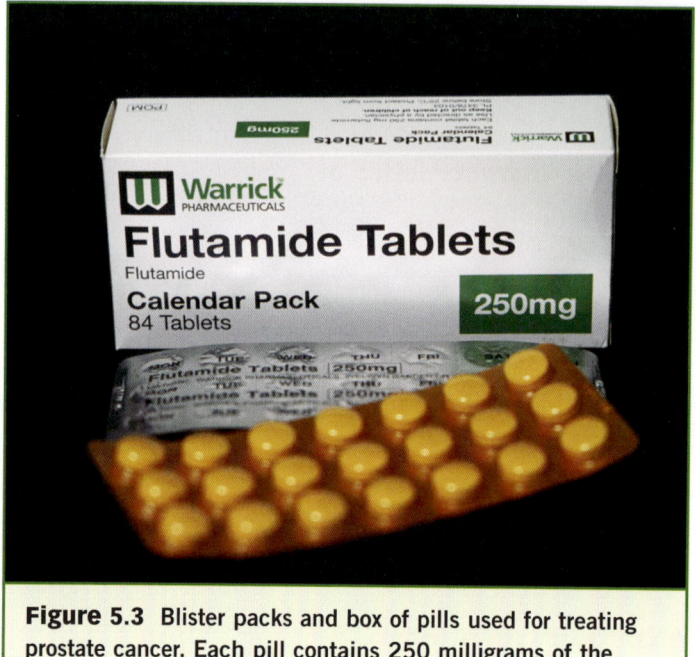

Figure 5.3 Blister packs and box of pills used for treating prostate cancer. Each pill contains 250 milligrams of the anti-androgen drug flutamide. © Joan Sher/Photo Researchers, Inc.

with a luteinizing hormone-releasing hormone (LHRH) for the treatment of metastatic cancer of the prostate. Nilutamide is approved for use in combination with surgical castration for the treatment of metastatic prostate cancer. Other treatments are preferred to using these drugs when possible, because they can cause the gradual development of female characteristics. These characteristics are described in greater detail in the next section on adverse effects. Each of these drugs are available as tablets or capsules for oral administration.

Adverse Effects of the Androgen Antagonists

Most of the unwanted effects of the androgen antagonists result from androgen activity being blocked in noncancerous tissues of the body. These drugs are only used to treat cancer in men, so the negative effects all relate to stopping the activity of male hormones, and the development of female sexual characteristics. The drugs are often given in combination with luteinizing hormone-releasing hormones (LHRH), which will be described in the next section. Treatment commonly results in hot flashes, decreased sexual desire and ability to perform sexually, general muscle aches and pains, changes in bowel habits, and swelling of breast tissue. These symptoms are reversible when the patient stops taking the drug if the patient did not have surgical **castration**. Another problem that can occur is a change in liver enzymes. Therapy often includes monitoring of these enzymes to avoid damage to the liver.

LUTEINIZING HORMONE-RELEASING HORMONE (LHRH) AGONISTS

Luteinizing hormone (LH) is released by the pituitary gland in the brain in response to a hormone called LH releasing hormone (LHRH). LHRH also stimulates the release of follicle-stimulating hormone (FSH) from the pituitary gland. Both LH and FSH circulate throughout the body and stimulate the appropriate tissues to produce estrogens and testosterone.

The LHRH agonists include goserelin, leuprolide, and triptorelin. When an LHRH agonist is first administered, the production of estrogens and testosterone is briefly stimulated because the drugs act like the body's own LHRH, but with longer dosing, the pituitary cells become desensitized to the drug, and hormone production falls to levels as low as when the ovaries or testicles are removed. This is useful when treating tumors whose growth is stimulated by the presence of these hormones.

Uses and Characteristics of the LHRH Agonists

The LHRH agonists are commonly used in combination with the antiandrogens to treat prostate cancer in men. They may also be used for the treatment of breast and endometrial cancers in women. These drugs are given as subcutaneous injections. Goserelin is used alone for the palliative treatment of advanced cancer of the prostate, and in combination with flutamide for treating locally confined prostate cancer prior to and during radiation therapy. It is also indicated for use in the palliative treatment of advanced breast cancer in pre-menopausal women and women who are very near menopause (perimenopausal). Leuprolide and triptorelin are indicated for the palliative treatment of advanced prostate cancer.

Adverse Effects of the LHRH Agonists

These drugs result in a decrease in the normal levels of hor-mones, and their adverse effects are similar to the adverse effects of the antiandrogen and antiestrogen drugs discussed earlier. Symptoms may include hot flashes, decreased sexual desire and ability to perform sexually, general muscle aches and pains, changes in bowel habits, swelling of breast tissue, occa-sional muscle weakness, fatigue, mood changes, joint and mus-cle aches and pains, nausea, and water retention. These symptoms are most often managed with supportive care, and by educating the patient to manage their activities to avoid making these symptoms worse.

ANDROGENIC AGONISTS

Only one androgenic agonist, fluoxymesterone, is used as a cancer drug. It has many of the effects that the natural andro-gens have on the body. At large enough doses, it suppresses the release of FSH from the pituitary gland just as the LHRH ago-nists do. Although it shares some of the same characteristics as the LHRH agonists, fluoxymesterone's activity against cancer is not well defined. In women, it can be useful in treating certain types of hormone-responsive breast cancer. It is also used to treat other noncancerous hormone disorders in men, in which their bodies do not produce enough testosterone.

Uses and Characteristics of Fluoxymesterone

Fluoxymesterone is used for the palliative treatment of recurrent androgen-responsive breast cancer in women who went through menopause more than one year ago but less than five years ago; or who have been proven to have a hormone-dependent tumor. The actual role of the male hormones in breast cancer is not as well understood as the role of the female hormones, however, in some breast cancers that respond to male hormones, fluoxymesterone is clearly effective.

Its use in women who are still experiencing menstruation is avoided when possible, because fluoxymesterone can cause masculine characteristics to develop and not all of them go away completely when the patient stops taking the drug. These characteristics are described further in the next section on adverse effects.

Adverse Effects of Fluoxymesterone

Fluoxymesterone can cause dangerous increases in circulating calcium (hypercalcemia) when it is used to treat patients with breast cancer. Hypercalcemia can cause dehydration, nausea, vomiting, muscle weakness, bone loss, and mental confusion, and can become fatal if it is not treated rapidly. Since calcium is excreted in the urine, measuring urine calcium levels regularly is a useful way to check for this problem. Fluoxymesterone can also damage the liver. Women taking this drug can experience virilization (development of masculine characteristics) of their bodies. Some of these symptoms include facial hair growth, deepening of the voice, and loss of menstrual periods. Other symptoms that are often experienced with this drug include upset stomach, vomiting, anxiety, depression, and acne.

6

Molecularly Targeted Agents

As described in Chapter 1, the process of cell growth and division is complex and is controlled by many different molecular processes. Greater understanding of the details of cell division unlocks the potential to find specific chemicals that can precisely and selectively act on only one controlling step. These steps are called molecular targets, and the drugs that interfere with them are called molecularly targeted agents, or molecular-target agents. In the treatment of cancer, these agents are designed to interfere only with molecular targets in cancer cells, leaving healthy cells untouched. Creating these kinds of specifically engineered agents is called "rational drug design." The class of molecularly targeted drugs is made up mainly of agents that were designed and created in the laboratory, although it also includes some naturally occurring substances whose anticancer activity was discovered, rather than engineered.

The first successful example of rational drug design was the creation of captopril, a high-blood-pressure drug that was approved for use in the United States in 1981. Captopril was created in the laboratory to inhibit an enzyme after the exact molecular structure of the enzyme was carefully determined. In the treatment of cancer, imatinib (brand name Glivec®, manufactured by Novartis) was the first successful example of this approach. Once the structure and role of an enzyme that is specifically active in chronic myelogenous leukemia (CML, a blood cancer) were identified, the search for a drug to inhibit the enzyme was on. American researcher, Dr. Brian Druker, recognized in the early 1990s while working for Novartis that imatinib was active, and started the long process of testing in the laboratory and in patients. In 2001, the drug was approved for use in the United States.

RETINOIDS

Retinoids are drugs related to vitamin A. They include bexarotene, tretinoin, and alitretinoin. Retinoids control normal cell growth, cell **differentiation** (the normal process of making cells different from each other), and cell death. Retinoids bind to receptors on the cell nucleus.

There are two major classes of retinoid nuclear receptors: retinoic acid receptors (RAR) and retinoid-X-receptors (RXR). Each of these types of receptors works differently in different tissues. The retinoid drugs each work by binding to different retinoid receptors. The newest retinoid drug, bexarotene, is specifically attracted to the RXR class of receptor and is sometimes called a rexinoid drug.

Uses and Characteristics of the Retinoids

Retinoids are a relatively new type of anticancer drugs. They have been used alone or in combination to treat a variety of cancers and have also been used in experiments to try to prevent certain types of cancer. Research on their role in both cancer treatment and prevention continues.

Table 6.1 The Retinoids

Generic Name	Trademarked name (manufacturer)
Bexarotene	Targretin® (Ligand Pharmaceuticals)
Tretinoin, ATRA	Vesanoid® (Roche)
Alitretinoin	Panretin® (Ligand Pharmaceuticals)

Tretinoin is used to treat a kind of blood cancer called acute promyelocytic leukemia (APL), in which the bone marrow produces a large number of immature blood cells and few or no mature cells. These immature cells cannot function normally. People with this cancer develop bleeding problems and immune system deficiencies. Tretinoin activates RAR receptors, causing the immature cells to mature. This, in turn, signals the bone marrow to stop producing immature cells. Although this treatment can help patients achieve **remission** (the decrease or disappearance of disease) of their symptoms, tretinoin must be used in combination with chemotherapy to eliminate the cancer cells in the bone marrow. Tretinoin is used to induce remission in patients with APL who failed to respond to or cannot use anthracycline-based chemotherapy, and is available in capsules.

Alitretinoin is a naturally occurring retinoid that binds to and activates all known retinoid receptors. Alitretinoin inhibits the growth of Kaposi's sarcoma (KS) when applied to affected areas of the skin. It is available as a topical (applied to the skin) gel, and is approved for use in the treatment of skin lesions in patients with AIDS-related Kaposi's sarcoma. It is not used when systemic therapy is required to treat Kaposi's sarcoma.

Bexarotene is a member of a subclass of retinoids that selectively activate retinoid X receptors (RXRs). These retinoid receptors have different functions in the cell than the retinoic acid receptors (RARs). Bexarotene binds and activates only the retinoid X receptors, which inhibits the growth of some tumor cells. It is approved to treat the skin lesions of cutaneous T-cell lymphoma in patients who failed to respond to at least one prior systemic therapy.

The Adverse Effects of the Retinoids

Retinoids are associated with skin problems such as dryness, itching, and sun sensitivity. They may also cause reversible increases in liver enzymes, temporary abnormal lipid levels, and low thyroid levels (**hypothyroidism**). Many of these symptoms are also caused by vitamin A overdose. In fact, taking vitamin A supplements while taking retinoids may make the adverse effects worse.

MONOCLONAL ANTIBODIES

Antibodies are proteins that specifically attach to and destroy cells and substances that are harmful to the body (**antigens**). These proteins are manufactured by cells of the body's immune system, and typically protect the body from bacteria, viruses, pollen, and other invading substances. The immune system also recognizes and destroys native cells of the body that are diseased or damaged. Scientists have taken advantage of this property by creating **monoclonal antibodies** that recognize proteins on the surface of cancerous cells.

Monoclonal antibodies, which include alemtuzumab, cetuximab, imatinib mesylate, trastuzumab, rituximab, bevacizumab, gemtuzumab ozogamicin, ibritumomab tiuxetan, and 131I-tositumomab, are produced in the laboratory from a single type of cell. They only recognize one antigen. Normal antibody-producing cells do not live very long and can only produce a limited number of antibodies. In order to mass-produce the antibody in the laboratory, one of these short-lived cells is fused to a fast-growing cancer cell that can live indefinitely. The resulting hybrid cell (**hybridoma**) reproduces rapidly and generates large quantities of highly specific antibody.

Since human immune cells are difficult to grow in the laboratory, scientists first used mouse hybridomas to produce antibodies. These antibodies often caused severe allergy-like reactions in the people who received them because of the presence of material from the mouse cells, so scientists combined part of the antibody-producing genes in mouse cells with similar genes from human cells. This produces a partly mouse-derived and partly human-derived antibody called a **chimeric** monoclonal antibody. This partly humanized protein has a

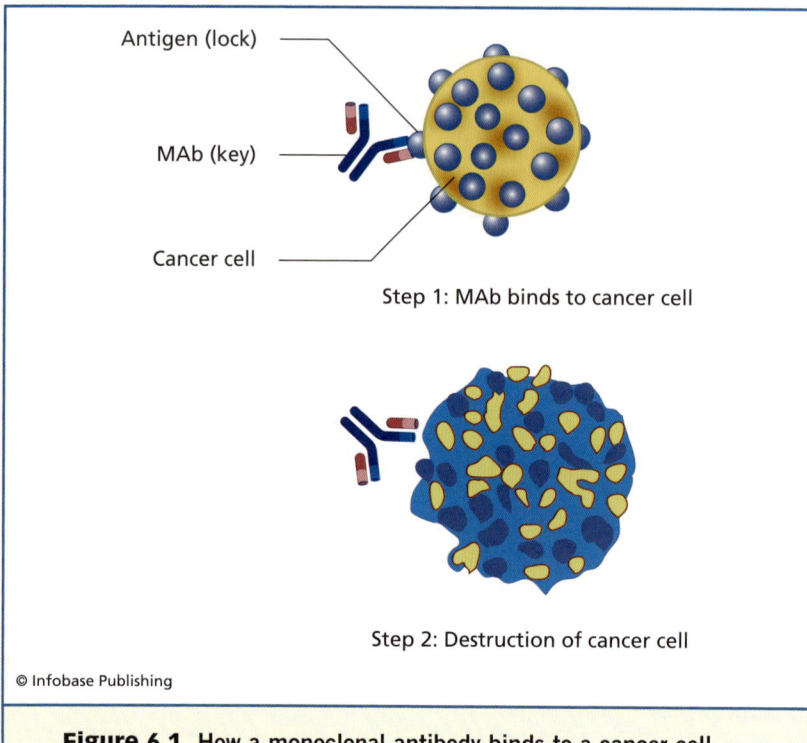

Antigen (lock)

MAb (key)

Cancer cell

Step 1: MAb binds to cancer cell

Step 2: Destruction of cancer cell

© Infobase Publishing

Figure 6.1 How a monoclonal antibody binds to a cancer cell.

better chance of not stimulating an allergy-like response in a patient.

Monoclonal antibodies are being researched for use in treating many diseases, including cancer. Some are given as pure antibodies, which act directly on cancer cells to destroy them. Others are **conjugated** (chemically bound) to drugs or radioactive agents, which are carried by the antibodies to the cancer cells where the chemical's destructive effects are limited to the tumor.

Unconjugated Monoclonal Antibodies

Alemtuzumab is an antibody directed against a protein called CD52 that is found on the surface of normal and malignant white blood cells. Although it can cause temporary bone

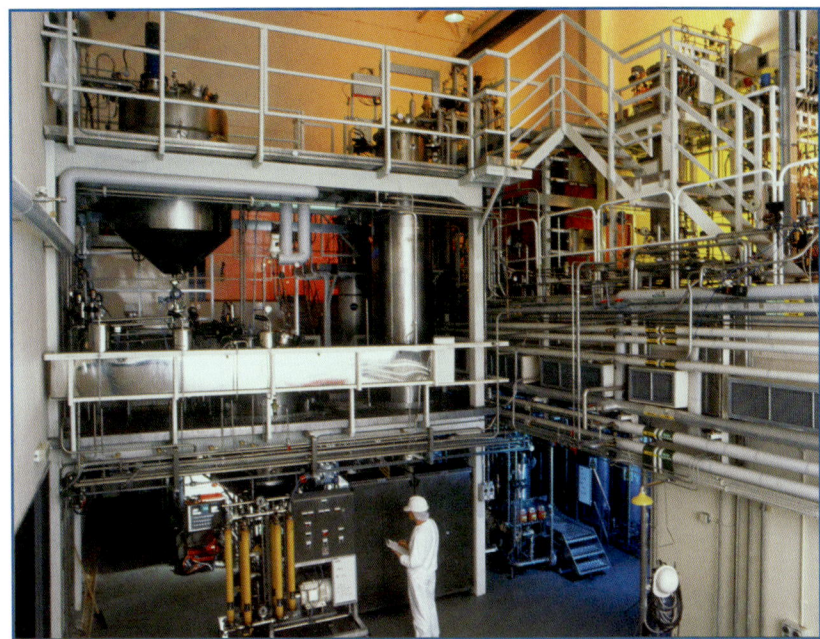

Figure 6.2 A large-scale fermenter used in the commercial production of monoclonal antibodies. © James Holmes/Cell Tech, Ltd./Photo Researchers, Inc.

marrow suppression because of its effects on normal cells, it is an effective agent in the treatment of a type of leukemia called B-cell chronic lymphocytic leukemia (B-CLL). B-cells, or B-lymphocytes, are immune system cells that produce antibodies when they mature.

Rituximab is directed against a cell surface protein on white blood cells called CD20. This protein appears on 90 percent of B-cell non-Hodgkin's lymphomas, as well as on normal immature and mature B-lymphocytes. CD20 does not appear in bone marrow stem cells or other normal cells, making rituximab a very specific agent against certain CD20-positive, non-Hodgkin's lymphomas.

Cetuximab binds and inhibits the epidermal growth factor receptor (EGFR) on cell surfaces. Some cancers produce large

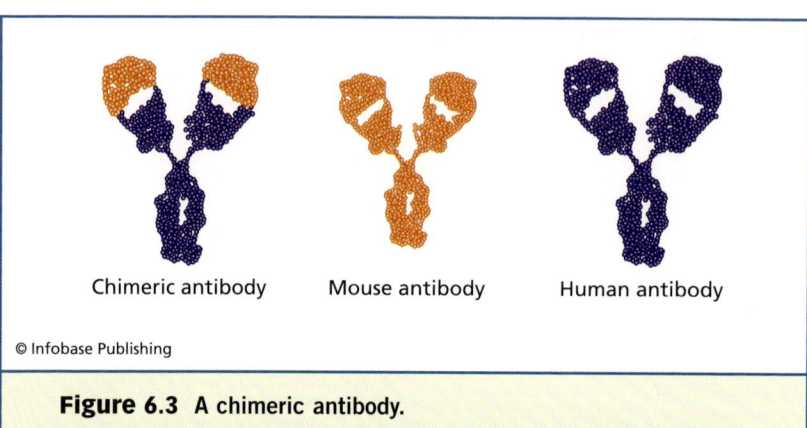

Chimeric antibody   Mouse antibody   Human antibody

© Infobase Publishing

Figure 6.3 A chimeric antibody.

quantities of this receptor (**overexpression**), making them sensitive to the presence of epidermal growth factor (EGF) so that they respond with renewed growth. Cetuximab is approved for the treatment of colorectal cancer, either alone or in combination with irinotecan.

Trastuzumab, like cetuximab, is specific for a cell surface growth factor receptor. It binds to a class of receptor known as HER2. This receptor is commonly overexpressed in 25 percent to 30 percent of breast cancers. A laboratory test can determine whether this receptor is present in a patient's tumor. Trastuzumab is approved for use alone or in combination with palitaxel in patients with HER2-positive breast cancer.

Bevacizumab binds to yet another growth factor receptor, vascular endothelial growth factor receptor (VEGFR). As a tumor grows larger, it outgrows the blood supply of the local, normal tissues and needs to develop its own blood supply to nourish its growing cells. The growth of new blood vessels is called **angiogenesis**, and it is stimulated as vascular endothelial growth factor (VEGF) binds to cells that line the blood vessel walls. Bevacizumab blocks VEGF from acting on these receptors, effectively starving the tumor. It is approved for use in combination with 5-fluorouracil for the treatment of metastatic colorectal cancer.

Table 6.2 The Monoclonal Antibodies

Generic Name	Trademarked name (manufacturer or distributor)
Alemtuzumab	Campath® (Berlex)
Cetuximab	Erbitux® (Bristol-Myers Squibb and ImClone)
Trastuzumab	Herceptin® (Genentech)
Rituximab	Rituxan® (Genentech)
Bevacizumab	Avastin® (Genentech)
Gemtuzumab ozogamicin	Mylotarg® (Wyeth)
Ibritumomab tiuxetan	Zevalin® (Biogen Idec)
131I-Tositumomab	Bexxar® (GlaxoSmithKline)

Conjugated Monoclonal Antibodies

Gemtuzumab ozogamicin is an antibody conjugated, or chemically bound to a cancer drug. The drug is an anticancer antibiotic called calicheamicin. The antibody binds to a cell surface protein called CD33, which is found on immature leukemic cells, on normal immature white blood cells, and on some bone marrow cells. This surface protein is found in more than 80 percent of patients with acute myeloid leukemia (AML). Gemtuzumab acts like a stealth bomber, secretly bringing death to the cell. When the antibody binds to CD33, the cell brings this surface protein inside itself, pulling the antibody and its calicheamicin along with it. Once inside the cell, calicheamicin is released where it binds to DNA molecules, breaking them and killing the cell. It is approved for use in CD33-positive AML in patients 60 years or older who are going through their first relapse after the start of treatment and who are not candidates for other chemotherapy.

Both ibritumomab tiuxetan and I-131 tositumomab are antibodies conjugated with radioactive substances. They are

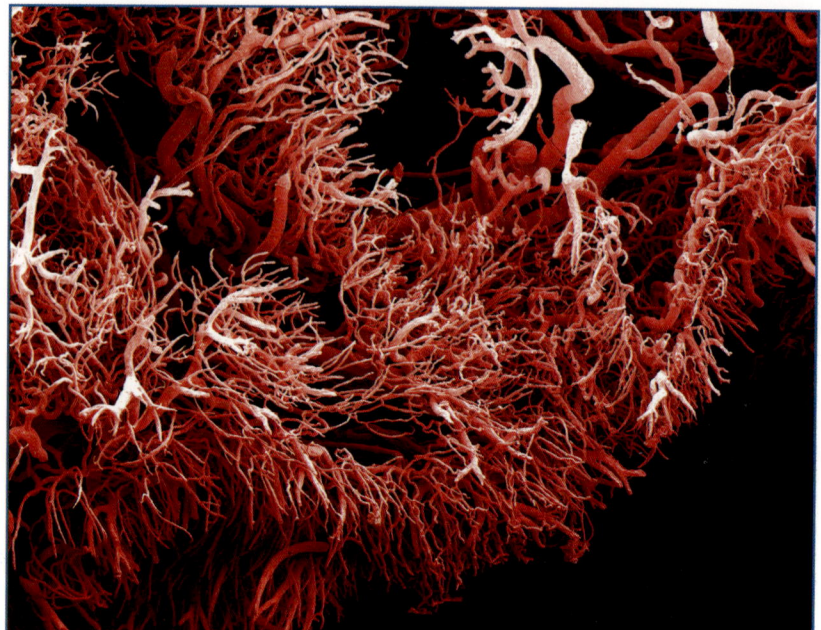

Figure 6.4 Colored scanning electron micrograph of a resin cast of blood vessels from an intestinal tumor. This branching network of vessels surrounded the tumor, supplying it with blood. © Clouds Hill Imaging Ltd./Photo Researchers, Inc.

sometimes referred to as radioimmunotherapeutic agents. Radiation therapy has been used successfully to treat many different cancers for many decades, but this treatment unnecessarily exposes a lot of healthy tissue to the effects of radiation. These drugs were developed to spare the healthy tissues as much as possible. Ibritumomab delivers radioactive yttrium (a metallic element) and radioactive indium (also a metallic element). Tositumomab delivers radioactive iodine. These radioactive substances were chosen for their relatively short half-lives, the time it takes for the radioactive energy to decrease by 50 percent. This is important both for limiting the amount of radiation delivered to the patient and for diminishing problems with excreting radioactive waste after dosing.

Because a patient excretes some radiation after receiving a dose, patients must exercise very careful hygiene to keep from exposing their family. However, the **half-life** for ibritumomab is so short that the radiation decreases to almost nothing shortly after dosing and the patient does not have to take any special precautions.

The antibodies in both drugs bind to the CD20 surface protein on B-cell non-Hodgkin's lymphoma, just as rituximab does. In fact, they are both approved to treat non-Hodgkin's lymphoma in patients who have relapsed after, or not responded to, rituximab treatment.

Dosing is very similar with both agents. In the case of tositumomab, patients first receive nonradioactive iodine. Because the thyroid gland normally absorbs iodine from the bloodstream, pretreatment saturates the thyroid gland with the element so it does not absorb any of the radioactive iodine from the therapy. After the first dose with the radioactive antibody, patients are scanned every few hours to measure the drug remaining in their body over time. Since everyone's metabolism is different, and patients excrete the drug at different rates, these scans are important to help determine the right dose for a particular patient for the rest of their treatments. Patients who receive tositumomab must follow careful rules about disposing their wastes, handling their laundry, and other hygiene, and physical contact with people for some days after their dosing, since the radiation from the iodine lasts a while and members of their family could be exposed if they contact any excreted drug.

Adverse Effects of Monoclonal Antibodies

Monoclonal antibody treatment for cancer is given intravenously, but is generally thought to have milder adverse effects than traditional chemotherapy. The adverse effects that occur are usually the result of the body reacting to the presence of the foreign antibody protein. The result is an allergic reaction and can include fever, chills, headache, nausea, vomiting, and rashes. These reactions can be severe, and even fatal, in some individuals, so careful observation of the patient is necessary during and after every infusion. Many of these drugs are given after pretreatment with antihistamines to prevent allergic complications.

Rituximab can act so rapidly and completely that some patients may experience tumor lysis syndrome, a reaction of the body's metabolism to the rapid breakdown of the tumor cells. Blood levels of potassium, uric acid, and phosphate can rise dangerously as levels of calcium fall well below normal. The reaction is serious and may be fatal, sometimes resulting in kidney failure. Early medical management is critical.

In addition to the allergic reactions typical of the monoclonal antibody drugs, cetuximab has occasionally caused pulmonary **edema** (an abnormal collection of fluid between the cells). More frequently, it produces an acne-like rash.

Congestive heart failure can occur in patients taking trastuzumab, so this drug is **contraindicated** (not recommended) for patients with heart problems.

Patients taking bevacizumab can experience problems with wound healing, minor and serious bleeding problems, thromboembolic events, and **hypertension** (high blood pressure). Bevacizumab's effect on blood vessels is related to the adverse effects unique to this monoclonal antibody.

Because gemtuzumab ozogamicin binds to normal immature white blood cells and even to some bone marrow cells, myelosuppression will occur. This drug has also been associated with infusion reactions, pulmonary edema, liver toxicity, and tumor lysis syndrome.

CONJUGATED PROTEIN

Conjugated protein, or denileukin diftitox, is made up of two proteins. Manufactured by Ligand Pharmaceuticals, it is sold under the brand name Ontak®. One protein comes from a toxin produced by the bacteria that causes the disease diphtheria. The other protein binds to a cell receptor called CD-25 on certain immune cells. These two proteins are fused to each other, so that when the one protein binds to the CD-25 receptor on a cell, it delivers the toxin to that cell. This drug literally carries a cell-killing poison directly to cancer cells, as long as the cancer cell has the CD-25 receptor. This is similar to the way some of the conjugated antibodies work, except that neither of the two proteins in this drug is an antibody. Certain types of lymphomas and leukemias carry this receptor, and denileukin diftitox is approved for use in lymphoma that produces the CD-25 receptor.

Uses and Characteristics of Conjugated Protein

Denileukin diftitox is used to treat patients with persistent or recurrent cutaneous T-cell lymphoma that produces the CD-25 receptor. It is administered as an IV infusion, usually for five consecutive days, every 21 days. This cycle is repeated until the disease goes into remission, but not usually more than four times.

Adverse Effects of Conjugated Protein

Serious allergic reactions can occur when these proteins are injected into the bloodstream, and when fluid and protein leak from the blood vessels into the tissues of the body. Most patients experience adverse effects that include flu-like symptoms, gastrointestinal problems (such as nausea, vomiting, and diarrhea), changes in heart rhythm and blood pressure, muscle aches and pains, neurotoxicity, skin rashes and itching, and coughing and breathlessness. White blood cell counts decrease in most patients, making them more susceptible to infections.

TYROSINE KINASE INHIBITORS

Tyrosine kinase inhibitors, which include imatinib mesylate, gefitinib, and erlotinib, are the newest class of anticancer drugs. They are sometimes called small-molecule tyrosine kinase inhibitors. As mentioned earlier, many cells, including cancer cells, have receptors on their surfaces for epidermal growth factor (EGF), a protein that the body normally produces to promote the growth and replication of cells. This property of growth promotion offers a key mechanism for interfering with the uncontrolled growth of cancer cells. When EGF attaches to epidermal growth factor receptors (EGFRs), it activates an enzyme called tyrosine kinase inside the cells. Tyrosine kinase triggers a cascade of chemical reactions that cause the cells to proliferate and spread. These small-molecule tyrosine kinase inhibitors enter the cell and block the tyrosine kinase enzyme. In this way, even when EGF binds to the receptor, the chemical cascade that triggers growth never gets started.

Uses and Characteristics of Tyrosine Kinase Inhibitors

Imatinib mesylate is used to treat certain types of chronic myeloid leukemia (CML) and a rare type of solid tumor of the digestive tract called a gastrointestinal stromal tumor (GIST).

Gefitinib is used to treat advanced non-small cell lung cancer that has failed to respond to platinum-based and docetaxel chemotherapies. Platinum-based cancer drugs include cisplatin and paraplatin and are described in Chapter 2. Docetaxel is a cancer drug derived from natural sources and is described in detail in Chapter 4.

Erlotinib is used to treat patients with locally advanced or metastatic non-small cell lung cancer treated with at least one prior chemotherapy regimen.

Adverse Effects of Tyrosine Kinase Inhibitors

Diarrhea, rash, and acne are common adverse effects of the tyrosine kinase inhibitors, and can become severe. Nausea, vomiting,

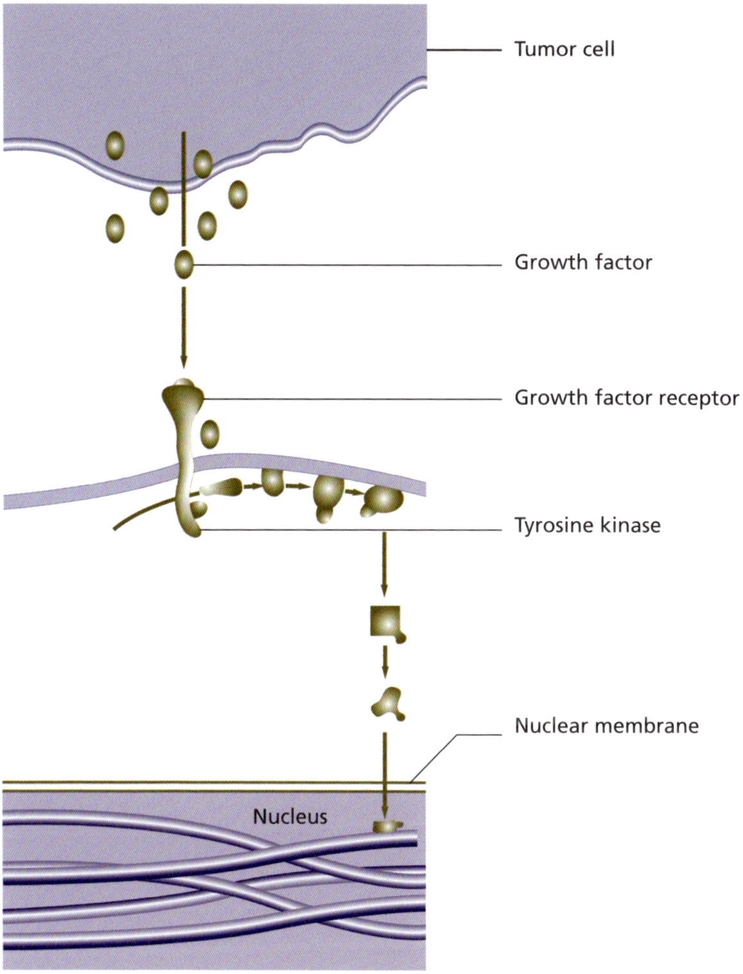

Tumor cell

Growth factor

Growth factor receptor

Tyrosine kinase

Nuclear membrane

Nucleus

© Infobase Publishing

Figure 6.5 Mechanism of action of the tyrosine inhibitors. Growth factors cause the production of tyrosine kinase, which stimulates cell growth. Tyrosine kinase inhibitors interfere with this process and inhibit the growth of cancer cells.

Table 6.3 The Tyrosine Kinase Inhibitors

Generic Name	Trademarked name (manufacturer or distributor)
Imatinib mesylate	Glivec® (Novartis)
Gefitinib	Iressa® (AstraZeneca)
Erlotinib	Tarceva® (OSI Pharmaceuticals and Genentech)

edema, fatigue, dry skin, itchy skin (pruritus), and muscle aches and pains are also typical effects of this class of drugs. These drugs are all metabolized in the liver, and they sometimes cause liver toxicities. Physicians may monitor the liver function of patients who take these drugs to avoid problems.

Imatinib shares the skin and digestive system effects of the other tyrosine kinase inhibitors, but the edema it causes can become severe and affect the heart, lung, and brain. Patients need to be monitored to identify any sudden fluid retention.

In a small number of patients, gefitinib therapy causes a kind of lung toxicity called interstitial lung disease (ILD). In ILD, the lung tissue is affected two ways: The walls of the air sacs in the lung become inflamed, and the **interstitium** (tissue between the air sacs) develops fibrosis, causing the lung to lose its elasticity. This can be fatal if not treated immediately.

Like gefitinib, imatinib is known to cause ILD, and patients need to be monitored for changes in coughing or breathlessness.

PROTEASOME INHIBITOR

Proteasomes are enzyme complexes that exist in all cells. They are part of the many tools that a cell uses to regulate its growth and life cycle. Specifically, proteasomes digest proteins or parts of proteins that regulate the cell cycle. Some of these proteins stop cell growth and some stimulate growth. Proteasomes destroy or activate some of these proteins through total or partial digestion. This activity maintains a balance of regulatory proteins for normal cell growth and death. Proteasomes in some types of cancer cells go into overdrive, rapidly digesting proteins and tipping the balance in favor of unregulated growth. The only proteasome inhibitor on the market today, bortezomib (sold under the brand name Velcade®), enters the cell and blocks this important enzyme complex, forcing cancer cells to reenter the cell cycle, ultimately ending in apoptosis. Bortezomib is given by intravenous injection. It is indicated for the treatment of multiple myeloma patients who have received at least one prior therapy.

Adverse Effects of the Proteasome Inhibitor

The most commonly experienced adverse effects seen with the use of proteasome inhibitor include generalized weakness, diarrhea and nausea, constipation, **peripheral neuropathy**, vomiting, fever, loss of appetite and weight, aches and pains, anemia, headache, and cough. Heart problems, including congestive heart failure, can occur with this drug.

7

Biologic Response Modifiers

In the 1890s, American surgeon William B. Coley was frustrated at the inability of surgery to cure cancer and searched the medical records to find an answer. He came across something that had been known for hundreds of years but was rarely used to try to cure cancer. Sometimes, people who caught an acute bacterial infection while they were suffering from a malignant cancer experienced a regression in their cancer. In fact, in 1868, an unnamed doctor deliberately infected a neck cancer patient with erysipelas, an infection of the skin by the bacterium *Streptococcus pyogenes*. He placed the patient in a ward that was known to have a high rate of erysipelas, and left the man there until he caught the infection. The patient eventually developed a fever and a full-blown case of erysipelas, after which his tumor shrank rapidly, but not completely. The tumor later recurred. Besides this case, Coley found other references to examples where erysipelas produced a more durable response in cancer patients.

Coley experimented with this infective approach to treating cancer. Eventually, he developed an injection of heat-killed bacteria that incorporated a combination of two bacteria: *Streptococcus pyogenes* and *Serratia marcescens*. This injection was eventually referred to as Coley's Toxins. Coley observed that the more severe the patient's response, the more successful the treatment was. He determined that the goal of therapy should be to produce a high fever and chills with each repeated dose. He continued to administer his treatment to thousands of cancer patients over the next 45 years of his medical career, collecting valuable information about tumor response to this assault on the immune system.

It is believed today that Coley's Toxins stimulates the body's production of immune system proteins that kill invading cells. The injection modified the immune system's natural defensive response. Coley's early work on using the body's native defense mechanisms against cancer is a forerunner of modern efforts to do the same, resulting in the development of clinically useful biologic response modifiers (BRMs). This chapter discusses the use of these BRMs that arise from modern science's sophisticated understanding of the body's immune system.

HOW DO BIOLOGIC RESPONSE MODIFIERS WORK?

The body's immune system relies on complex interactions between many organs and cells in the body. The immune system creates cells and proteins that directly attack antigens and unwanted body cells and also creates chemical messengers that mobilize other parts of the immune system for the attack. These chemical messengers are referred to collectively as **cytokines**. Interferons and interleukins are types of cytokines that have been exploited to artificially modify the body's response to the presence of cancer cells.

Interferons (IFN) were the first cytokines produced in the laboratory. There are three major types of interferons: interferon alpha, interferon beta, and interferon gamma. The IFNs have antiviral activities, and can affect the metabolism, growth, and maturation of cells. Interferon alpha is most widely used to treat cancer.

Interleukins (IL) are a large collection of proteins that are involved in cell-to-cell communication. They have many functions, but mainly they direct other immune cells to grow and differentiate. Of all the interleukins, IL-2 is most effective against cancer.

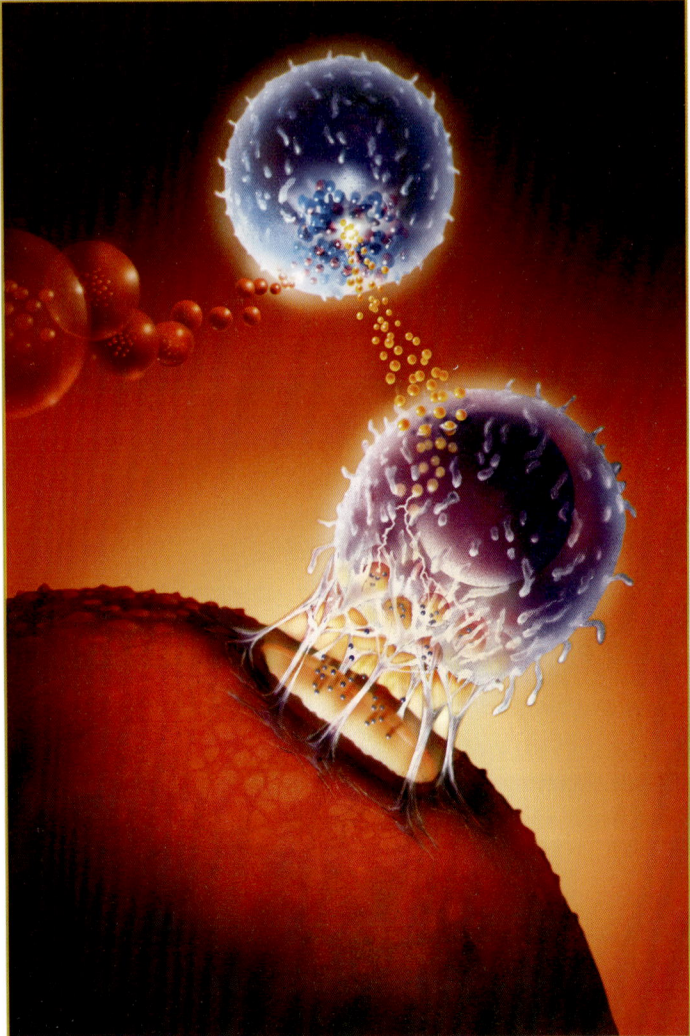

Figure 7.1 The body's immune response to a cancer cell. Clockwise from the middle left: Cytokine type 2 messengers (orange) stimulate a helper T cell (blue) to release type 1 cytokines, which in turn activate the killer T cell (lavender), which in turn seeks to destroy the cancer cell. The killer T cell punctures and poisons the cancer cell (bottom). Type 2 cytokines are released by either B cells or dendritic cells.© Jim Dowdalls/Photo Researchers, Inc.

Another way to use the immune system against cancer is to administer a substance that, like Coley's Toxins, mobilizes the immune system in a nonspecific way, but unlike Coley's Toxin, is directed only against the affected tissue. A substance called BCG live is used in this way. It will be discussed separately from the interferons and interleukins.

USES AND CHARACTERISTICS OF BIOLOGIC RESPONSE MODIFIERS

In addition to treating a viral infection of the liver, hepatitis C, IFN-alpha-2a is approved for use in treating two kinds of leukemia: chronic myelogenous leukemia and hairy cell leukemia. IL-2 is approved to treat metastatic renal cell carcinoma (a kidney cancer) and metastatic melanoma (a skin cancer). These drugs are given by intravenous injection.

ADVERSE EFFECTS OF BIOLOGIC RESPONSE MODIFIERS

Interferons are used to treat a variety of illnesses, so the adverse events experienced by a patient may depend on the underlying disease being treated. Generally, treatment with interferon-alpha causes flu-like symptoms (fever, chills, and muscle aches), diarrhea, nausea, vomiting, headache, depression, sleep disturbances, cough, difficulty breathing, heart rhythm changes, hair loss, rash, sweating, and dry and itchy skin. Signs of depression and other psychiatric changes may be particularly important to watch for, and this drug should be avoided in people with already-existing psychiatric problems. In addition, interferon-alpha causes severe bone marrow suppression and can cause serious damage to structures in the eye. All patients should be monitored closely when taking this drug.

Interleukin-2 can have profound effects on lung and heart function and should only be used in people who did not have lung or heart disease. It also impairs white blood cell function, leading to increased vulnerability to infections. In some

Table 7.1 The Biologic Response Modifiers

Generic Name	Trademarked name (manufacturer or distributor)
Interferon alfa-2a, recombinant	Roferon-A® (Roche Pharmaceuticals)
Interleukin-2 (IL-2, aldesleukin)	Proleukin® (Chiron Corporation)
BCG live	TheraCys® (Sanofi Aventis); TICE BCG® (Organon)

patients, interleukin-2 can cause plasma protein and fluid to leak out from the bloodstream into the tissues, resulting in serious circulatory problems and even death. More commonly, interleukin-2 therapy causes the same adverse effects as interferon-alpha.

BCG LIVE

Bacillus Calmette-Guérin contains a weakened strain of the organism that causes tuberculosis. A form of this preparation is sometimes used to vaccinate people against this disease. BCG can be administered into the bladder to treat certain types of bladder cancer. In the bladder, it promotes a local acute inflammatory reaction that eventually causes the formation of **granulomas** (small nodules of constantly inflamed tissue). The exact mechanism of action is unknown, but the antitumor effect appears to depend on the action of the white blood cells that are attracted to the granulomas.

BCG can rarely cause an active tuberculosis infection. More commonly, in addition to the flu-like symptoms caused by other biologic response modifiers, BCG treatment may cause frequent, painful urination, and blood in the urine.

8

Miscellaneous Agents

In this chapter, several drugs that are difficult to categorize will be introduced. They are hard to group with other drugs mostly because their precise anticancer mechanism cannot be explained, but also because their chemical structures do not fit in with the types of agents already discussed. They have, however, proven to be useful in the treatment of cancer, some of them for many decades.

This chapter will also look at agents that are commonly used to help patients stay on therapy. As previous chapters demonstrated, many chemotherapies and biological therapies are difficult to tolerate, causing adverse effects that can cut a treatment cycle short. The supportive agents described here are used to help alleviate these effects so that patients can get the maximum benefits from their prescribed therapy.

ASPARAGINASE

Asparaginase is an enzyme extracted from intestinal bacteria that breaks down asparagine, an amino acid that normal body cells easily manufacture from nutrients and use to support a variety of cellular functions. The cancer cells in some types of acute leukemia, especially lymphocytic leukemia, are unable to make their own asparagine, and must get their supply from normal cells. By administering asparaginase to patients with this kind of cancer, the circulating supply of the amino acid is depleted, literally starving the

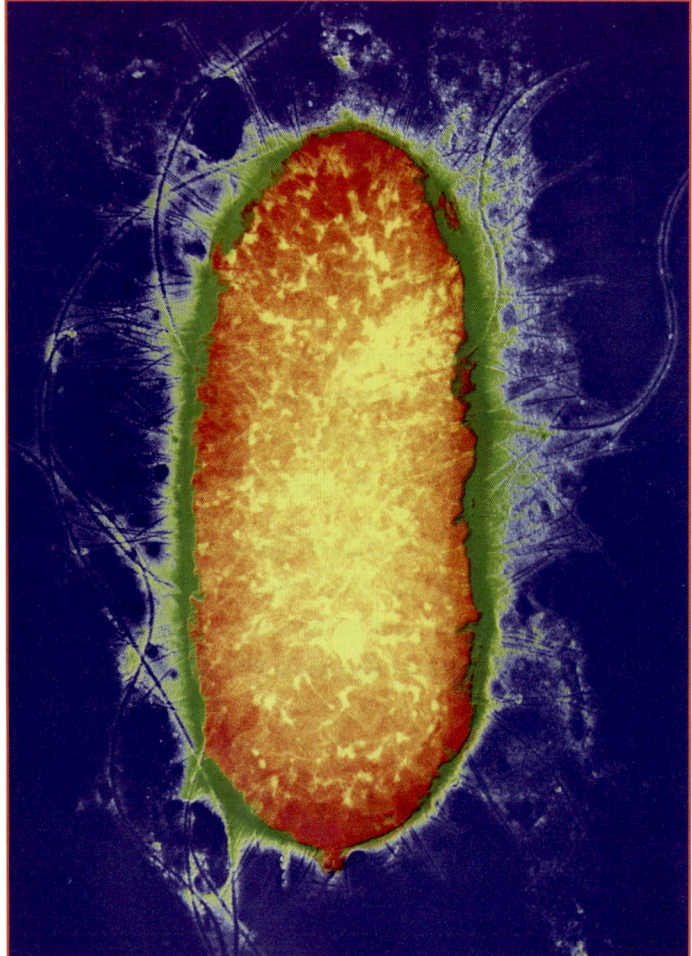

Figure 8.1 Erwinnia chrysanthemi. In the laboratory this bacteria is grown for the enzyme L-asparaginase that it contains. The enzyme is extracted and purified as a drug for acute lymphoblastic leukemia (ALL), a cancer of the white blood cells found mainly in children. © A. B. Dowsett/Photo Researchers, Inc.

Some thyroid tumors seem to grow in response to TSH. The thyroid hormones levothyroxine and liothyronine are synthetic versions of naturally occurring thyroid hormones. They can be given to patients to keep levels of circulating thyroid hormone high and suppress the release of TSH from the pituitary. These drugs are usually used as adjunctive therapy to radiation and surgery. Without TSH, these tumors are unable to keep growing. These drugs are available as tablets and as an injection.

HYDROXYUREA

Hydroxyurea is sometimes classified as an antimetabolite, although its mechanism against cancer is not well defined. Laboratory experiments suggest that hydroxyurea interferes with the replication of DNA without stopping the production of protein. It seems to make cells more susceptible to the effects of radiation, possibly by making it hard for the cell to repair radiation damage. The inability to make repairs eventually kills the affected cells. Significant tumor response to hydroxyurea has been demonstrated in melanoma, resistant chronic myelocytic leukemia, and recurrent, metastatic, or inoperable carcinoma of the ovary.

Bone marrow suppression, and the immune system problems that accompany it, can occur in patients who receive hydroxyurea. In addition, patients may experience gastrointestinal symptoms (such as nausea, vomiting, and diarrhea), and skin problems, including discoloration, rash, and ulceration.

Hydroxyurea, used together with irradiation therapy (delivery of radiation from a source placed inside the body) is used in the local control of primary squamous cell carcinomas of the head and neck, except for the lip. It is available in capsule form for oral administration.

ARSENIC TRIOXIDE

Exactly how arsenic trioxide works to kill cancer cells is not clear, but in the laboratory, it causes the kind of DNA fragmentation seen in cells that die off as part of their normal cell cycle (apoptosis). Some patients treated with arsenic trioxide have experienced symptoms similar to a syndrome called APL (acute promyelocytic leukemia) differentiation syndrome, including fever, dyspnea, weight gain, and fluid imbalances in the lung. This syndrome can be fatal, but it can be managed with high doses of dexamethasone, one of the glucocorticoids discussed earlier in this chapter, often without needing to stop the anticancer therapy. Arsenic trioxide can also cause serious changes in heart rhythm and congestive heart failure. Most patients experience some drug-related toxicity, most commonly **leukocytosis** (an increase in the number of white blood cells in the bloodstream), nausea, vomiting, diarrhea, abdominal pain, fatigue, edema, hyperglycemia, dyspnea, cough, rash or itching, headaches, and dizziness.

PROCARBAZINE

Procarbazine appears to interfere with protein, DNA, and RNA synthesis in cells, and it has proven to be useful in combination therapy. Currently, its only approved use is in combination therapy for advanced stages of Hodgkin's disease.

This orally administered drug commonly causes nausea and vomiting, which can be managed in part by starting out with low doses that are divided up during the day for the first week, before increasing the dose to therapeutic levels.

ALTRETAMINE

Although the chemical structure of altretamine resembles the structure of the alkylating agents (discussed in Chapter 2), laboratory studies did not reveal similar activity. How this drug works to treat cancer is still unknown, but it is active in certain forms of ovarian cancer.

Altretamine is indicated for use as a single agent in the palliative treatment of patients with ovarian cancer that persists or recurs after therapy with a cisplatin or alkylating agent–based combination. It is available in capsules for oral administration.

Altretamine commonly causes myelosuppression, neurotoxicity (including symptoms such as mood disorders, disorders of consciousness, **ataxia** [lack of coordination], dizziness), and nausea and vomiting.

ARSENIC—THE GOOD AND THE BAD, THE UPS AND THE DOWNS

Arsenic has a history of therapeutic use over 2,000 years long. It also has a long history of use as a deadly poison. Because a large dose of arsenic causes symptoms similar to those of the disease cholera, it was a popular way for the wealthy to eliminate their rivals during the Middle Ages, when cholera was common. Some historians believe that French Emperor Napoleon Bonaparte was slowly killed with arsenic slipped into his wine after his exile to the island of Elba.

On the other hand, solutions of arsenic trioxide were used to treat a variety of disorders—including hypertension, bleeding ulcers, and rheumatoid arthritis—throughout the 18th, 19th, and early 20th centuries. In 1910, the organic arsenic compound Salvarsan was developed to treat syphilis. It was the first effective treatment discovered for this sexually transmitted disease.

Observations made in the late 1800s showed that arsenic solutions decreased the number of circulating white blood cells. As a result, arsenic trioxide was used as a treatment for leukemia until the advent of radiation therapy in the early 1900s. Arsenic trioxide rose in popularity again in the 1930s when it was found to be effective in treating chronic myelogenous leukemia after radiation therapy. This treatment was later replaced as chemotherapeutic agents were discovered. In the late 1990s, Chinese researchers reported great success using arsenic trioxide in the treatment of acute promyelocytic leukemia (APL). In 2000, the FDA approved the use of arsenic trioxide for the treatment of certain genetic types of relapsed or refractory APL.

PORFIMER

Porfimer falls into a unique category among anticancer drugs. It is a photosensitizing (causes cells to become sensitive to light) agent that prepares cells for photodynamic (causing a toxic reaction to light) therapy. It binds to a variety of cells and tissues when injected into the body. For two days after the injection, normal cells get rid of the porfimer, but tumor cells retain it. Then, a laser light is directed at the cancer cells using a very thin glass strand called an optic fiber. Exposure to the light alters the chemical, probably releasing **free radicals** (reactive atoms or groups of atoms that are missing an electron), which kill the tumor cells. Porfimer is approved for use to relieve obstruction from cancers of the esophagus or bronchial tubes of the lung, and to treat certain lung cancers.

Although most normal cells of the body can eliminate porfimer, it tends to remain in the skin and eyes. For as long as three months after injection, patients should protect themselves from exposure to light by wearing hats, sunglasses, and appropriate clothing. Sunblock lotions only block ultraviolet (UV) radiation, so they do not provide effective light protection. Exposure to the sun or any bright light source may cause blistering of the skin or damage to the eyes. In addition, patients may experience some pain and irritation near the tumor site.

DRUGS THAT SUPPORT ANTICANCER DRUG THERAPY

This section provides a brief summary of the many different agents used to alleviate the adverse events of cancer treatment. In addition to the agents listed here, supportive therapy for cancer patients can include a wide range of drugs to treat other problems associated with the illness, such as poor appetite, susceptibility to infection, or disabling pain.

MYELOID AND ERYTHROID STIMULATING FACTORS

Many of the anticancer agents in this book decrease the production of blood cells because one of their effects is bone marrow suppression. This is unavoidable for many anticancer drugs. Chemotherapy is designed to kill cells that are actively dividing, and this includes some normal cells as well as the cancerous ones. Bone marrow is constantly dividing and producing the cells that will eventually develop into the many different cells that circulate in the bloodstream. Until the development of bone marrow stimulating factors, chemotherapy had to be interrupted, changed, or stopped altogether when marrow suppression became severe. Of course, for cancers like leukemia in which the bone marrow overproduces certain blood cells, bone marrow suppression may play an important role in successful therapy.

Bone marrow suppression can cause many problems for the patient. Not having enough white blood cells can leave the patient susceptible to infections and unable to fight them off if they do get infected. If the patient has too few red blood cells, he or she becomes anemic and unable to adequately transport oxygen and other nutrients throughout the body. Without enough platelets in the bloodstream, the patient may bleed too easily and excessively, since platelets start forming a clot at the site of blood vessel injury.

The bone marrow stimulating factors discussed here are biologic response modifiers. They boost the body's natural processes and help them to recover from damage. Each substance specifically boosts the production of a certain type of cell, and is chosen based on a given patient's needs. With careful planning and a rapid response to changes in patient blood counts, doctors can continue to administer the most effective anticancer therapies at the necessary doses by providing the kind of boost their patient's bone marrow needs. In addition, these drugs are often used after bone marrow

Table 8.2 Myeloid and Erythroid Stimulating Factors

Generic Name	Trademarked name (manufacturer or distributor)
Epoetin	Epogen® (Amgen)
	Procrit® (Ortho Biotech)
Darbepoetin alfa	Aranesp® (Amgen)
Oprelvekin	Neumega® (Wyeth)
Filgrastim	Neupogen® (Amgen)
Pegfilgrastim	Neulasta® (Amgen)
Sargramostim	Leukine® (Berlex)

transplant therapy, which is performed to treat certain leukemias and lymphomas. Bone marrow transplant involves first destroying the bone marrow with chemotherapy, then replacing it with healthy bone marrow. This new bone marrow benefits from the added stimulation of these biologic response modifiers.

All of these drugs are given by injection, often subcutaneously. Blood cell counts are monitored carefully throughout the course of therapy.

Epoetin and darbopoetin alfa are man-made versions of human erythropoietin (EPO). EPO is produced naturally in the body, mostly by the kidneys, and stimulates the bone marrow to produce red blood cells. Epoetin and darbopoetin are used to prevent or treat anemia caused by AIDS, surgery, chronic kidney disease, or cancer. In addition to these agents, the body needs iron to make red blood cells, so patients might be instructed to take iron supplements and other vitamins to improve iron absorption while they are on this therapy. Since it takes the body about six weeks to produce a measurable response to epoetin or darbopoetin treatment, preventing anemia in cancer patients requires coordinated timing with anticancer therapy.

These are very effective therapies, but like any treatment, they have risks. They sometimes cause convulsions, especially during the first 90 days of treatment. They may also increase the risk of blood clots, so patients should be alert for signs of chest pain or shortness of breath. Some patients may develop antibodies to epoetin or darbopoetin, causing a lack of red blood cells called pure red cell aplasia (PRCA). This requires an immediate discontinuation of treatment. These problems are not frequently seen, however. More commonly, patients may develop less dangerous symptoms, such as high blood pressure, joint pain, headache, or nausea.

Oprelvekin is a synthetic version of the cytokine interleukin-11 (IL11). IL11 stimulates the body to produce platelets, which are a critical part of blood clotting. It takes five to nine days of daily dosing with oprelvekin to start increasing platelet levels in the bloodstream. Reduced platelets are a common adverse effect of platinum-based drugs and the alkylating agents, and a common reason for interrupting these therapies or decreasing the doses of these agents.

A common adverse effect of oprelvekin therapy is edema, which can cause problems with breathing, vision, or heart function. On occasion, these problems may be serious. More often, patients may experience heart arrhythmias, cough, rhinitis (runny nose), sore throat, nausea, vomiting, or diarrhea.

Filgrastim and pegfilgrastim are different synthetic forms of human granulocyte colony-stimulating factor (G-CSF). G-CSF is normally produced by many cells in the body. It stimulates the bone marrow to produce a kind of white blood cell called a neutrophil. Without neutrophils, the body is very vulnerable to infections. Filgrastim or pegfilrastim treatment of patients receiving anticancer therapy that suppresses white

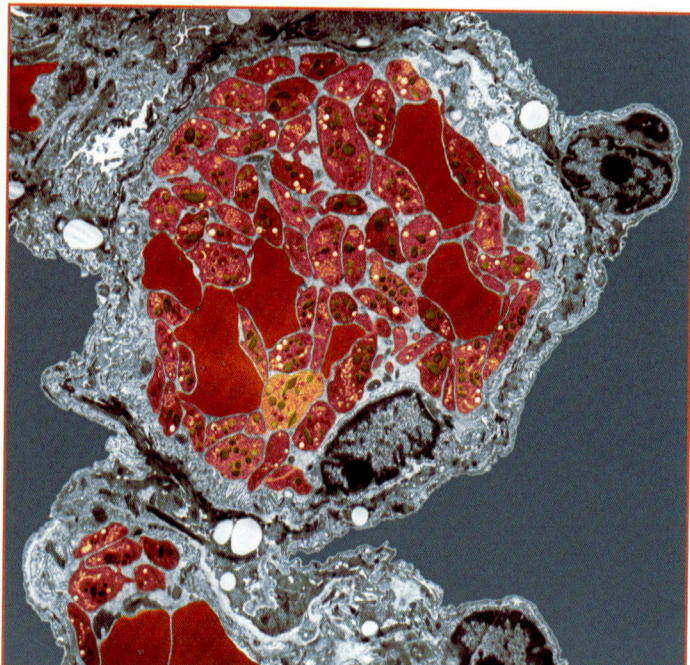

Figure 8.2 Active platelet. Platelet cells are formed in the bone marrow and circulate in blood in large numbers. © A. B. Dowsett/Photo Researchers, Inc.

blood cells reduces the number of infections and the use of antibiotics in these patients.

Both of these agents work the same way, but pegfilgrastim is designed to stay in the body longer, reducing the need for frequent doses. Allergic reactions have occurred in patients receiving these drugs and, rarely, rupture of the spleen. Less serious adverse effects included nausea, vomiting, diarrhea, hair loss, and bone pain.

Sargramostim is a man-made form of the naturally occurring protein granulocyte macrophage-colony stimulating factor (GM-CSF). GM-CSF is produced by the immune system and stimulates the formation of white blood cells, including granulocytes and macrophages, which take part in inflammatory

Table 8.3 The Biosphonates

Generic Name	Trademarked name (manufacturer or distributor)
Pamidronate	Aredia® (Novartis)
Zoledronic acid	Zometa® (Novartis)

reactions. In addition, GM-CSF induces the production of neutrophils. Sargramostim is given to stimulate the production of white blood cells and neutrophils. The most common adverse effects while taking sargramostim are fever, weakness, chills, headache, nausea, diarrhea, and muscle and bone pain.

BISPHOSPHONATES

Certain cancers are more likely to metastasize to the bone than others, and when they do, they can cause a condition called hypercalcemia of malignancy. Bone is the largest storage site of calcium in the body. When cancer spreads to the skeleton, bone tissue starts to break down. This causes calcium levels in the blood to rise dramatically, resulting in damage to kidneys, nerves, brain, and other tissues and organs. The biphospho-nate drugs pamidronate and zoledronic acid prevent the breakdown of bone tissue and the resulting release of calcium into the bloodstream. Kidney damage is an uncommon adverse effect of using these drugs, as is osteonecrosis (death of bone tissue) of the jaw. More commonly, patients experi-ence a flu-like syndrome after treatment, along with nausea, vomiting, or diarrhea.

CYTOPROTECTIVE AGENTS

The cytoprotective agents, which include amifostine, dexrazox-ane, and mesna, are used to protect normal cells from damage by anticancer drugs. Anticancer therapy poses many risks to healthy cells. Usually, the damage done to the healthy cells cannot be avoided. If the damaging action were blocked, then the anticancer activity would be blocked as well. In some cases, however, certain healthy tissues are singled out for damage by the anticancer drug in a specific way. This specificity is the key to finding protective agents. Not many such agents exist yet, and the need for them may decrease as the anticancer drugs themselves become more cancer-specific, sparing healthy cells.

Mesna was already discussed in Chapter 2. It is administered with ifosfamide to protect the cells of the bladder. The metabolites of ifosfamide are excreted in the urine, and can damage the lining of the bladder if mesna is not also present.

Amifostene is a drug designed to protect the kidneys from cisplatin. Kidney damage is a serious adverse effect of cisplatin therapy. Amifostene is given 30 minutes before the cisplatin dose to give it time to reach the kidneys, where it binds to the toxic metabolites of cisplatin and makes them harmless. Amifostene is also useful in protecting healthy tissues from damage during radiation therapy for cancer.

After long dosing with doxorubicin, cardiac toxicity is inevitable. Giving dexrazoxane to a patient who has already taken doxorubicin and needs to take more can reduce the incidence and severity of cardiomyopathy (heart muscle damage). The actual mechanism of action of dexrazoxane is not known. It is only useful if it is administered 30 minutes before the dose of doxorubicin.

Table 8.4 Cytoprotective Agents

Generic Name	Trademarked name (manufacturer or distributor)
Mesna	Mesnex® (Bristol-Myers Squibb)
Amifostene	Ethyol® (MedImmune Oncology)
Dexrazoxane	Zinecard® (Pfizer)

9

The Future

Although doctors have been trying to treat cancer for thousands of years, rigorous scientific methods for developing and proving effective therapies really only came into use a little over 100 years ago. Starting in the late 1800s, advances in growing cells in the laboratory, understanding cancer-causing agents, diagnosing illness with new techniques, and using chemotherapy to treat diseases all contributed to the birth of the science of oncology. Early treatments used a sledgehammer approach, applying toxic agents in hard-to-tolerate doses and regimens. Patients suffered through nausea, vomiting, infections, and other problems with little or no treatment for these effects. Few people survived the cancer or its treatment.

As the life processes of normal and cancerous cells become better understood, whole new approaches to destroying cancer were discovered. With the understanding of the genetic basis of life and the intricate machinery that guides cell replication and growth came insight into clever ways to put that machinery out of order. This gave rise to drugs that attacked DNA, broke delicate cellular structures, and blocked cells from receiving critical nutrients and growth signals. As scientists learned more about the body's own defensive mechanisms, they developed ways to manipulate the immune system to make it work harder and to mimic its methods by creating "souped-up" antibodies that could destroy cancers that the body could not destroy on its own. In addition to new drugs, innovative ways to deliver therapy have been crafted. With each new wave of knowledge, cancer therapy has become more specific, more potent, and more successful. Over the past 10 years, death rates in the United States from breast, stomach, prostate, colon and rectum, and uterus cancers have steadily declined. A diagnosis of cancer is no longer the death sentence it once was.

Sometimes, understanding cancer and the mechanisms of its treatment has helped scientists identify better methods of delivering old drugs to take advantage of their useful properties. A good example of this is liposomal doxorubicin. Liposomes are artificially created microscopic droplets of the same fatty material, called phospholipid, that makes up most cell membranes. These droplets were originally created as a drug-delivery mechanism, and liposomal doxorubicin successfully puts this idea into practice. The liposome protects healthy cells from some of the toxic effects of doxorubicin, while also keeping the drug circulating in the blood longer, so that more doxorubicin reaches the cancer cells. This approach has reduced the incidence of cardiac problems, nausea, and hair loss that are typical of doxorubicin therapies. Liposomal delivery systems are also being researched for other chemotherapies. In addition, the use of liposome technology itself is continually being refined. For example, work is currently being done to try to create heat-sensitive liposomes that will only release drugs in tissues that are heated to a certain temperature.

The idea of packaging a toxic drug safely for delivery to its site of action has inspired a lot of research. From protein and lipid molecules to microscopic spheres of plastic or other artificial materials, safe wrappers for toxic drugs that will also deliver the contents specifically to cancer cells are actively under investigation.

Another interesting delivery approach approved in recent years is a small wafer that is saturated with carmustine. This product, called the Gliadel Wafer®, is manufactured by MGI Pharma. These wafers are designed to be implanted directly into certain types of brain tumor, where they slowly release the drug.

There are two big advantages to this approach: The drug is only released where it is needed, which limits the adverse effects, and the drug can be delivered directly to the tumor in the brain. Getting drugs to brain tissue is often difficult because the blood circulation of the brain does not allow drugs through the blood vessel walls the way the blood in the rest of the body does. This blood-brain barrier makes it difficult to deliver many therapies to the brain. The wafer is the first marketed delivery device of its kind in anticancer therapy. Work continues to look for other substances that can be saturated with a drug and placed directly where needed. Such materials are already being used successfully to treat diseases of the eye and blood vessels of the heart.

Variations on this theme are also being pursued. Slow-release materials, including plastic, mineral, and organic molecules that can be implanted into the body, may make directed delivery a standard form of therapy administration someday. Coupling these materials with technologies that allow controlled release are on the cutting edge of drug delivery research. Complex solutions to the problem of controlled release include delivering drugs from injectable microprocessors, similar to those that, in larger versions, control computers. Simpler methods involve storing the drug in an iron-rich material, injecting it into the bloodstream, and attracting the material to the intended site with magnets. The possibilities are only limited by imagination.

There are many different cellular mechanisms that are vulnerable to attack by anticancer drugs. More such mechanisms come to light regularly as research delves deeper into the complex processes of a cell's life. It would be beyond the scope of this book to list and describe the hundreds of cell features and mechanisms that have been identified as potential cancer drug targets. Each year, new tools for examining the details of cellular functions are discovered and applied in creative ways. With each advance, new enzymes, proteins, growth controlling factors, genes, and other cell components are defined.

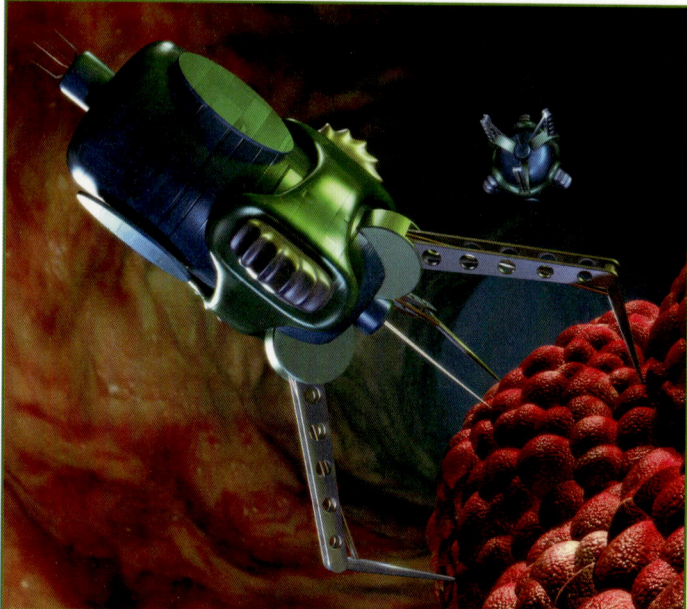

Figure 9.1 Medical nanorobot. Computer artwork of a nanorobot injecting a drug into a cancer (red) in a human body. This is an example of a possible future application of microscopic robot technology to treat disease. © Roger Harris/Photo Researchers, Inc.

Processes that were once thought to be well defined turn out to be only part of a much bigger picture.

In the newest approaches to eliminating cancer, medical science merges its new understanding of the cancer cell with the ability to create and manipulate genetic material. The goal is to beat cancer at its foundation—the DNA of the cell. While many chemotherapy agents already break, bind, and otherwise interfere with DNA strands, the newest approaches attempt to rewrite the DNA code to either end the cancer cell's life or give it a more normal function. Whether delivered through the use of innovative materials as discussed above, manufactured antibodies, or, by using a man-made virus, the right bits of genetic code could change the future of cancer treatment.

Glossary

acute—Short-term.

advanced disease—Cancer that returns, is inoperable, or spreads to other parts of the body.

agonist—A drug that produces the same action as the substance it mimics.

alkylating agents—Chemicals that disrupt cellular DNA by adding short organic molecules (alkyl groups) to DNA bases, changing the way DNA molecules bond, or causing mispairing of DNA bases, ultimately causing cell death.

alopecia—Loss of hair.

analog—A chemical that is structurally similar to, but slightly different from, another chemical.

angiogenesis—The growth of new blood vessels.

anorexia—Prolonged loss of appetite.

antagonist—A chemical that opposes the action of another chemical.

antigen—Any substance that stimulates the immune system to respond by trying to remove or eliminate it.

anti-inflammatory—Anything that acts to relieve the redness, pain, and swelling typical of an inflammation, the body's response to certain types of injury.

apoptosis—Also called "programmed cell death," this is the natural process of cell death that ends with the dead cell being "cleaned up" by enzymes and other cells that specialize in removing waste materials.

arrhythmia—Disrupted beating of the heart that could lead to heart damage or even death if left untreated.

ataxia—Unsteadiness or lack of coordination. This could be a sign of damage to the muscles or the brain.

base—In DNA, a base is one of four nitrogen-containing molecules that are strung together in long, paired strands and define the genetic code.

benign—Noncancerous.

carcinoma—Cancer that grows from epithelial tissue, which is tissue that makes up the outer and inner linings of the body. Carcinomas account for as much as 90 percent of all cancers.

cardiac—Having to do with the heart.

cardioprotective—Referring to the substances that keep the heart safe from certain kinds of damage.

castration—Removal of the testicle; some drugs can temporarily block the male hormones so completely that even when the testicles are present, their action is referred to as chemical castration.

Glossary

catheter—A thin tube inserted into blood vessels or body cavities that allows a drug to be delivered or a sample to be removed

centrioles—Specialized tubular support structures that organize the division of cells.

chimeric—An antibody protein produced by a cell that has some human genes and some animal genes.

chronic—Long-term.

cirrhosis—Scarring and disrupted function of the liver.

conjugated—Chemically bound or joined.

contraceptives—Pregnancy preventatives.

contraindicated—Not recommended. Most drugs are not recommended for use under certain conditions, and these contraindications guide a doctor's prescribing decisions.

cytokine—Proteins that are used by the immune system to send chemical messages to other cells in the immune system.

cytoplasm—The watery fluid in the cell that surrounds its structures.

differentiate—To mature and develop into a specific form and function.

DNA (deoxyribonucleic acid)—The double-stranded, twisted molecule in the nucleus of a cell that carries the genetic code.

edema—The abnormal accumulation of fluid in the tissues of the body. It can impair the function of some organs, such as the heart.

endoplasmic reticulum—A cell structure that is important to protein synthesis.

erythrocyte—Red blood cell.

excision—When something is cut out, or surgically removed.

extravasation—When an injected drug leaks out of the vein and enters the local tissues during an intravenous injection. With some cancer drugs, this can cause irritation and damage to local tissues.

fibrosis—Formation of inflexible scar tissue. This can affect the normal function of some organs, such as the lungs.

first-line therapy—The first therapeutic regimen given to a newly diagnosed patient; this is followed by second-line therapy if the first attempt fails.

free radical—Atoms or groups of atoms that are missing an electron, which makes them chemically reactive. Free radicals in a cell can damage its structures and functions.

gastrointestinal system—The stomach and intestines.

granuloma—Small nodule of constantly inflamed tissue.

half-life—For radioactive materials, this is the amount of time it takes for 50 percent of the radiation to disappear.

hand-foot syndrome—Blistering and peeling of the hands and the feet caused by some cancer drugs.

homeostasis—The normal balance of growth and death. Cancer cells escape the normal restraints of homeostasis, allowing them to grow uncontrollably.

hybridoma—A cell that is fused to another type of cell; the fused cell has the properties of the original cells.

hyperpigmentation—Overproduction of the proteins that provide color to the skin.

hypertension—High blood pressure.

hypothyroidism—Decreased production of thyroid hormones.

immunosuppression—Inhibition of immune system functions that can result in greater susceptibility to infection.

induction therapy—Treatment whose goal is to start reducing the cancer in preparation for further treatment.

interstitium—In the lung, these are the cells and tissues between the air sacs.

intraarterial—Into an artery.

intrathecally—Into the membrane surrounding the spinal cord and brain and containing spinal fluid.

intravenous—In the vein.

intravenous infusion—Slow administration of a drug directly into a vein.

leukemia—This type of cancer is also called liquid cancer or blood cancer, and starts in the bone marrow. Leukemia typically causes overproduction of white blood cells that do not reach their mature form, but can also affect the production of red blood cells.

leukocyte—Any of several types of white blood cells.

leukocytosis—Overproduction of white blood cells.

lipid—Fatty or waxy chemicals. Lipids are an important part of cell membranes.

liposome—An artificially created microscopic droplet of the same fatty material that makes up most cell membranes. It is used to enclose a drug for safe delivery to its site of action.

lymphatic—Produced by or relating to the lymph system or lymph tissues (such as the spleen, lymph nodes, and tonsils). Lymphatic tissues are an important part of the immune system.

lymphocyte—Immune system cell that matures in and circulates through the lymph nodes and vessels; a type of white blood cell.

Glossary

lymphoma—Cancer that originates in the organs and tissues of the lymphatic system, including lymph nodes, spleen, or tonsils. Since lymph vessels circulate throughout the body, a lymphoma may develop in the lymph system of any organ, such as the stomach, breast, or brain.

lysosome—Sac of enzymes found in a cell.

malignant—Cancerous.

menopause—A time in a woman's life when her menstrual cycles stop and hormone production in her body changes.

metabolism—All the processes in the cell that provide energy and process materials for vital activities.

metastatic—Referring to cancer that appears in a part of the body that is away from where it originally started. The new sites are called metastases. This usually indicates an advanced stage of cancer.

microtubules—Hollow, tubular filaments of the protein tubulin. They provide structural support for the cell and play a role in separating cells during cell division.

mitochondria—An energy-producing structure in the cell.

monoclonal antibody—An immune system protein (antibody) that is produced from exact copies of a single cell.

mucositis—Inflammation of the mucous membranes found in the mouth, gastrointestinal system, and other organs of the body.

myeloma—Cancer that develops in the plasma cells of the bone marrow. The plasma cells produce some of the proteins that circulate in the bloodstream.

myelosuppression—Decreased function of the bone marrow, resulting in too few red and white blood cells being made; this can lead to a high risk of getting an infection and little chance of fighting the infection off.

neuropathy—Degeneration or damage to the nerves.

nitrogen mustards—A group of chemically related compounds that were originally developed for military use; they cause blistering of the skin, eyes, and lungs. Their effect on rapidly dividing cells in the blood and immune system led to their use in treating cancer.

nucleic acids—DNA and RNA, which can be found in the nucleus of the cell.

nucleus—The structure in the cell that stores the genetic material.

organelles—Specialized structures in the cell, like the organs in the body.

osteoporosis—A disease in which the bones lose their mass and become brittle and porous. This can be the result of slow loss of calcium over many years as occurs in response to hormonal changes in older women, or it can occur as a result of some cancers, lack of physical activity, or some drug treatments.

overexpression—Cellular overproduction of a protein.

palliative—A measure taken to ease symptoms without curing the disease.

peripheral neuropathy—Nerve damage or degeneration that occurs in the hands or feet and in the areas close to them, in the peripheral areas of the body. This painful condition can result from disease processes or as an adverse reaction to a drug.

pleura—A membrane that lines the abdominal cavity, heart, and lungs.

pleural effusion—Accumulation of fluid in the membranes that surround the lungs, heart, and abdomen. Fluid accumulation in these membranes can impair breathing and blood circulation.

prodrug—A drug that has to be chemically altered by the body in order to have a therapeutic effect.

pulmonary—Having to do with the lungs.

radiation therapy—A cancer treatment that uses concentrated beams of energy, like X-rays, to kill cancer cells.

receptors—Specialized proteins that latch onto specific molecules in the cellular environment and cause some change to happen in the cell as a result.

refractory—Refers to a disease that is resistant to therapy.

regimen—A systematic plan of therapy. In the case of cancer therapy, this could include a plan to administer several drugs or other therapies (like radiation or surgery) in a coordinated schedule.

remission—A decrease in, or disappearance of, disease, but not a cure.

renal—Having to do with the kidney.

ribosome—Small structure in the cell found on the endoplasmic reticulum that is necessary for manufacturing proteins.

sarcoma—Cancer that develops in supportive and structural body tissues, like bones, muscles, tendons, cartilage, and fat.

subcutaneously—Under the skin.

telomerase—An enzyme in immature cells that replaces the telomere after cell division, allowing the cell to keep dividing. Normal mature cells stop producing this enzyme, which limits the number of times they divide; some cancer cells keep producing it.

telomere—A structure at the end of the DNA strands that shortens each time a mature cell divides. When the telomere is gone, the cell stops dividing.

Glossary

thromboembolic—Causing a piece of a blood clot in a vessel to break away and block blood flow.

topically—On the surface of the skin.

toxicity—A poisonous or harmful effect of a drug.

transcription—The transfer of the genetic information in DNA; this must occur before the cell can make a copy of the DNA for when the cell divides.

tubulin—The protein that makes up microtubules, which form the structural support of the cell.

Antman, Karen H. "The History of Arsenic Trioxide in Cancer Therapy." *The Oncologist* 6 (2001): 1–2.

Bentor, Yinon. "Chemical Element.com—Iodine." Chemical Elements.com. Available online. URL: http://www.chemicalelements.com/elements/i.html. Downloaded on August 11, 2005.

Bickels, Jacob, Yehuda Kollender, Ofer Merinsky, and Isaac Meller. "Coley's Toxin: Historical Perspective." *Israel Medical Association Journal* 4 (2002): 471–472.

Biotech. "Cyberbotanica: Plants and Cancer Treatments." University of Texas Institute for Cellular and Molecular Biology. Available online. URL: http://biotech.icmb.utexas.edu/botany/. Downloaded on August 10, 2005.

Cancer Research, Treatment. "Who was Sidney Farber?" Dana Farber Cancer Institute. Available online. URL: http://www.dana-farber.org/abo/history/who/. Downloaded on July 21, 2005.

DeVita, V. T., S. Hellman, and S. A. Rosenberg. *Cancer, Principles & Practice of Oncology*, 7th ed. Philadelphia: Lippincott Williams & Wilkins, 2005.

Goodman, L. Sanford, J. G. Hardman, L. E. Limbird, and A. G. Gilman. *Goodman & Gilman's the Pharmacological Basis of Therapeutics*, 10th ed. New York: McGraw-Hill, 2001.

Lane, Sharon. "Cancer History." Rare Cancer Alliance. Available online. URL: http://www.rare-cancer.org/history-of-cancer.html. Downloaded on August 10, 2005.

Love, Richard R., and John Philips. "Oophorectomy for Breast Cancer: History Revisited." *Journal of the National Cancer Institute* 94, 19 (2002): 1433–1434.

Minton, Susan E. "New Hormonal Therapies for Breast Cancer." *Cancer Control* 6 (1999): 247–255.

Old, Lloyd. "Human Cancer Immunology." Memorial Sloan-Kettering Cancer Center. Available online. URL: http://www.mskcc.org/mskcc/html/11099.cfm. Downloaded on July 17, 2005.

Segota, Ena, and Ronald M. Bukowski. "The Promise of Targeted Therapy: Cancer Drugs Become More Specific." *Cleveland Clinic Journal of Medicine* 71 (2004): 551–560.

Skeel, Roland T. *Handbook of Cancer Chemotherapy*, 6th ed. Philadelphia: Lippincott Williams & Wilkins, 2003.

Urological Sciences Research Foundation. "Charles B. Huggins." University of Chicago Hospitals & Health Systems. Available online. URL: http://www.usrf.org/news/010308-huggins.html. Downloaded on August 27, 2005.

Bibliography

U.S. Food and Drug Administration. "A Brief History of the Center for Drug Evaluation and Research." Center for Drug Evaluation and Research. Available online. URL: http://www.fda.gov/cder/about/history/default.htm. Downloaded on June 14, 2005.

———. "History of the FDA." FDA History. Available online. URL: http://www.fda.gov/oc/history/default.htm. Downloaded on June 17, 2005.

Further Reading

Gifford, Rebecca. *Cancer Happens: Coming of Age With Cancer*, 1st ed. Sterling, VA: Capital Books, 2003.

Keene, Nancy, Wendy Hobbie, and Kathy Ruccione. *Childhood Cancer Survivors: A Practical Guide to Your Future*, 1st ed. Cambridge, MA: O'Reilly, 2000.

Web Sites

The Biology Project. "Cell Biology." University of Arizona. Available online at http://www.biology.arizona.edu/cell_bio/cell_bio.html.

Chembytes e-zine. "Nature's Bounty." The Royal Society of Chemistry. Available online at http://www.chemsoc.org/chembytes/ezine/2001/cragg_jan01.htm.

The Chemical Heritage Foundation. "Magic Bullets: Chemistry vs Cancer." Pharmaceutical Achievers. Available online at www.chemheritage.org/educationalservices/pharm/chemo/readings/ages.htm.

Index

Index

ethyleneimines, 26, 31–33
etoposide phosphate, 60–63
excision, 48, 118
exemestane, 66, 68
  adverse effects of, 72
  as aromatase inhibitor, 69
  indications for, 71
extravasation of anthra-cyclines, 60

Farber, Sidney, 38–39
fibrosis, 118
  pulmonary, 60, 92
filgrastim, 100, 108, 109–110
first-line therapy, 118
  irinotecan in, 61
floxuridine, 41, 44
fludarabine, 41, 45, 47
fluorodeoxyuridine (flox-uridine), 41, 44
fluorouracil, 41, 44
  with bevacizumab, 84
fluoxymesterone, 66, 76–77
flutamide, 66, 73–75, 76
folic acid, 38, 40–43
follicle-stimulating hor-mone, 75
Food and Drug Administration, 32, 35
frankincense (Boswellia thurifera), 49
free radicals, 106, 118
fulvestrant, 66, 68
  adverse effects of, 72
  as antiestrogen, 69
  indications for, 71
future trends in cancer therapy, 113–116

Galen (Roman doctor), 48
gastrointestinal system, 118

antimetabolites affecting, 47
gefitinib, 89–92
gemcitabine, 41, 44–45
gemtuzumab ozogamicin, 81, 85, 88
genes, 25
ginger root extract, 10
glucocorticoids, 101
goserelin, 66, 75–76
granulocyte colony-stim-ulating factor, 109–110
granulocyte macrophage-colony stimulating fac-tor, 110–111
granuloma, 118
  in BCG therapy, 98
Greece, ancient, plant-derived medicines in, 52

hairy-cell leukemia, 47
half-life of radioactive materials, 87, 119
hand-foot syndrome, 36, 119
heart problems, 117
  from antibiotic anti-cancer agents, 59–60, 112, 114
  from monoclonal antibody therapy, 88
  from taxanes, 55
HER2 and trastuzumab actions, 84
hexamethylmelamine, 26
Hippocrates, 10
histological classification of cancer, 20
historical aspects of can-cer drugs and therapy, 10
  alkylating agents in, 22–23
  antimetabolites in, 38–39
  arsenic trioxide in, 105

biologic response modifiers in, 94–95
  hormone therapies in, 64
  natural products in, 48–49
homeostasis, 12, 119
hormone therapies, 18, 21, 64–77
  androgen antagonists in, 73–75
  androgenic agonist fl oxymesterone in, 76–77
  available preparations for, 66
  historical aspects of, 64
  luteinizing hormone releasing hormone agonists in, 75–76
  mechanism of action, 65–67
  progestins in, 72–73
  in prostate cancer, 65, 73–74, 76
  selective estrogen receptor modulators in, 67–72
Huggins, Charles, 65
hybridoma, 81, 119
hydroxyurea, 100, 103
hypercalcemia
  from fluoxymesterone, 77
  of malignancy, bispho-sphonate therapy in, 111
hyperpigmentation, 119
  from bleomycin, 60
hypertension, 119
  from monoclonal antibody therapy, 88
hypothyroidism, 119
  from retinoids, 81

ibritumomab tiuxetan, 81, 85–87

Index

Index

Trademarks

Adriamycin is a registered trademark of Adria Laboratories; Alimta is a registered trademark of Eli Lilly and Company; Alkeran is a registered trademark of GlaxoSmithKline; Aranesp is a registered trademark of Amgen; Aredia is a registered trademark of Novartis; Arimidex is a registered trademark of AstraZeneca; Aromasin is a registered trademark of Pfizer; Avastin is a registered trademark of Genentech; Bexxar is a registered trademark of GlaxoSmithKline; BiCNU is a registered trademark of Bristol-Myers Squibb; Blenoxane is a registered trademark of Bristol-Myers Squibb; Busulfex is a registered trademark of ESP Pharma; Campath is a registered trademark of Berlex; Camptosar is a registered trademark of Pfizer; Casodex is a registered trademark of AstraZeneca; CEENU is a registered trademark of Bristol-Myers Squibb; Cerubidine is a registered trademark of Bedford Labs; Cosmegen is a registered trademark of Merck; Cytoxan is a registered trademark of Bristol-Myers Squibb; Doxil is a registered trademark of Ortho Biotech; DTIC-DOME is a registered trademark of Bayer Pharmaceuticals; Eligard is a registered trademark of Sanofi Aventis; Ellence is a registered trademark of Pfizer; Eloxatin is a registered trademark of Sanofi Aventis; Elspar is a registered trademark of Merck & Co., Inc.; Epogen is a registered trademark of Amgen, Inc.; Erbitex is a registered trademark of Bristol-Myers Squibb and ImClone; Etopophos is a registered trademark of Bristol-Myers Squibb; Ethyol is a registered trademark of MedImmune Oncology, Inc.; Eulexin is a registered trademark of Schering-Plough; Fareston is a registered trademark of Orion Corp.; Faslodex is a registered trademark of AstraZeneca; Femera is a registered trademark of Novartis; Fludara is a registered trademark of Berlex Laboratories; FUDR is a registered trademark of Roche; Gemzar is a registered trademark of Eli Lilly and Company; Gliadel is a registered trademark of Guilford Pharmaceuticals; Glivec is a registered trademark of Novartis; Halotestin is a registered trademark of Pfizer; Herceptin is a registered trademark of Genentech; Hexalen is a registered trademark of MGI Pharma; Hycamtin is a registered trademark of GlaxoSmithKline; Hydrea is a registered trademark of Bristol-Myers Squibb; Idamycin is a registered trademark of Adria Laboratories; Ifex is a registered trademark of Bristol-Myers Squibb; Iressa is a registered trademark of AstraZeneca; Leukeran is a registered trademark of GlaxoSmithKline; Leukine is a registered trademark of Berlex; Leustatin is a registered trademark of Ortho Biotech Products, L.P.; Lupron is a registered trademark of TAP Pharmaceuticals; Matulane is a registered trademark of Sigma-Tau Pharmaceuticals; Megace is a registered trademark of Bristol-Myers Squibb; Mesnex is a registered trademark of Bristol-Myers Squibb; Myleran is a registered trademark of GlaxoSmithKline; Mylotarg is a registered trademark of Wyeth; Mustargen is a registered trademark of Merck; Mutamycin is a registered trademark of Bristol-Myers Squibb; Navelbine is a registered trademark of GlaxoSmithKline; Neosar is a registered trademark of Sicor Labs; Neulasta is a registered trademark of Amgen; Neumega is a registered trademark of Wyeth; Neupogen is a registered trademark of Amgen, Inc.; Nilandron is a registered trademark of Sanofi Aventis; Nipent is a registered trademark of SuperGen; Nolvadex is a registered trademark of AstraZeneca; Novantrone is a registered trademark of Serono Pharmaceuticals; Oncovin is a registered trademark of Eli Lilly and Company; Ontak is a registered trademark of Ligand Pharmaceuticals; Panretin is a registered trademark of Ligand Pharmaceuticals; Paraplatin is a registered trademark of Bristol-Myers Squibb; Photofrin is a registered trademark of Axcan Pharma Inc.; Prempro is a registered trademark of Wyeth; Procrit is a registered trademark of Ortho Biotech; Proleukin is a registered trademark of Chiron Corporation; Prokine is a registered trademark of Immunex; Provera is a registered trademark of Pfizer; Purinethol is a registered trademark of GlaxoSmithKline; Rituxin is a registered trademark of Genentech; Roferon-A is a registered trademark of Roche Pharmaceuticals; Rubex is a registered trademark of Bristol-Myers Squibb; Sandostatin is a registered trademark of Novartis; Tarceva is a registered trademark of OSI Pharmaceuticals and Genentech; Targretin is a registered trademark of Ligand Pharmaceuticals; Taxol is a registered trademark of Bristol-Myers Squibb; Taxotere is a registered trademark of Sanofi Aventis; Temodar is a registered trademark of Schering-Plough; Thera-Cys is a registered trademark of Sanofi Aventis; TICE BCG is a registered trademark of Organon; Trelstar is a registered trademark of Watson Pharma, Inc.; Trisenox is a registered trademark of Cephalon Oncology; Valstar is a registered trademark of Anthra Pharmaceuticals and Medeva Pharmaceuticals; Velban is a registered trademark of Eli Lilly and Company; Velcade is a registered trademark of Millennium Pharmaceuticals; Vepesid is a registered trademark of Bristol-Myers Squibb; Vesanoid is a registered trademark of Roche; Vumon is a registered trademark of Bristol-Myers Squibb; Xeloda is a registered trademark of Roche; Zanosar is a registered trademark of Sicor Pharmaceuticals; Zevalin is a registered trademark of Biogen Idec; Zinecard is a registered trademark of Pfizer; Zoladex is a registered trademark of AstraZeneca; Zometa is a registered trademark of Novartis.

About the Author

Judith Matray-Devoti received her undergraduate degree in Pharmacy at the Ernest Mario School of Pharmacy, Rutgers University, and her Ph.D. in Physiology and Neurobiology, also at Rutgers University. She worked for a major pharmaceutical company for 17 years, starting out in toxicology research and moving on to managing medical information for the oncology and HIV franchises. Most recently, as medical director for medical communications companies, she has written, edited, and directed the creation of instructional materials for sales representatives, physicians, other healthcare professionals and pharmaceutical company executives and managers in a variety of therapeutic areas, especially cancer. She is a member of the American Medical Writers Association, American Pharmaceutical Association, and Mensa and lives in southern New Jersey.

About the Editor

David J. Triggle is a University Professor and a Distinguished Professor in the School of Pharmacy and Pharmaceutical Sciences at the State University of New York at Buffalo. He studied in the United Kingdom and earned his B.Sc. degree in Chemistry from the University of Southampton and a Ph.D. degree in Chemistry at the University of Hull. Following post-doctoral work at the University of Ottawa in Canada and the University of London in the United Kingdom, he assumed a position at the School of Pharmacy at Buffalo. He served as Chairman of the Department of Biochemical Pharmacology from 1971 to 1985 and as Dean of the School of Pharmacy from 1985 to 1995. From 1995 to 2001 he served as the Dean of the Graduate School, and as the University Provost from 2000 to 2001. He is the author of several books dealing with the chemical pharmacology of the autonomic nervous system and drug-receptor interactions, some 400 scientific publications, and has delivered over 1,000 lectures worldwide on his research.